Special Praise for *The Family Caregiver's Manual*

"I've known David Levy for quite some [...] saying he is clearly the subject-matter expert in family care[...] families I know who have worked with David sing his praise [...] to both his knowledge and his compassion. The information o[...] pages will be transformative to those who read it and need the skills and suggestions offered. I highly recommend this book."

Scott Greenberg
CEO ComForcare Senior Services, Author of the
award-winning book *Oh My God I'm Getting Older and So Is
My Mom* and host of a weekly radio show by the same name

"David Levy has been doing 'caregiving' since before that term was in vogue. In this book, David shares his wealth of knowledge. *The Family Caregiver's Manual* can be a lifesaver and is certain to engender a higher quality of life for all who will be touched by this knowledge."

Scott M. Solkoff, Esq.
Founder of Solkoff Legal, Florida bar
board-certified specialist in elder law

". . . a valuable tool that can assist and support unpaid family caregivers in their efforts to provide an improved quality of life for their loved ones while they maintain balance in their own lives. Educating family caregivers allows them to be better prepared to face the myriad issues that arise in caregiving."

Charles T. Corley
Former Secretary, Florida Department of Elder Affairs

"David Levy has made an impressive contribution to caregiving with the comprehensive material in *The Family Caregiver's Manual*. He skillfully and artfully helps the caregiver to answer questions of 'what if' in caregiving. His practical experience along with his masterfully crafted checklists and guides make this a must-read for everyone regardless of whether or not they are currently a caregiver."

Christopher J. Metzler, PhD
President/CEO of FHW Fit and FHW Squared
AARP Thought Leader

The
Family Caregiver's
Manual

The Family Caregiver's Manual

A Practical Planning Guide to Managing the Care of Your Loved One

David Levy

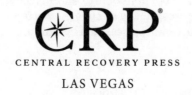

CENTRAL RECOVERY PRESS

LAS VEGAS

Central Recovery Press (CRP) is committed to publishing exceptional materials addressing addiction treatment, recovery, and behavioral healthcare topics.

For more information, visit www.centralrecoverypress.com.

Publisher: Central Recovery Press
            3321 N. Buffalo Drive
            Las Vegas, NV 89129

21 20 19 18 17 16   1 2 3 4 5

Library of Congress Cataloging-in-Publication Data

Names: Levy, David, (Gerontologist) author.
Title: The family caregiver's manual : a practical planning guide to managing
  the care of your loved one / David Levy.
Description: Las Vegas, NV : Central Recovery Press, 2016. | Includes
  bibliographical references and index.
Identifiers: LCCN 2016000456 (print) | LCCN 2016010896 (ebook) | ISBN
  9781942094128 (paperback) | ISBN 9781942094128 ()
Subjects: LCSH: Family social work. | Home nursing. | Care of the sick. |
  Caregivers. | BISAC: FAMILY & RELATIONSHIPS / Abuse / Elder Abuse. |
  REFERENCE / Personal & Practical Guides. | LAW / Elder Law. | MEDICAL /
  Long-Term Care.
Classification: LCC HV697 .L48 2016 (print) | LCC HV697 (ebook) | DDC
  649.8--dc23
LC record available at http://lccn.loc.gov/2016000456

Photo of David Levy by Paul Vattiato. Used with permission.

Cover design by The Book Designers
Interior design and layout by Deb Tremper, Six Penny Graphics

To Family Caregivers Everywhere

This manual was created to support all those who have been, are, or will be unpaid family caregivers. Understanding how to ascertain realistic options in an ever-changing and increasingly more detached system is critical for all family caregivers. My hope is that with the help of this manual, you will be able to understand those options more clearly and be enabled to make wiser decisions. It is also my hope that this manual will help you attain the one goal my efforts place foremost: gaining the peace of mind that comes from knowing that as a family caregiver, you did the best you could with what you had at the time you had to do it.

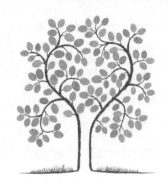

Table of Contents

Preface

Development of *The Family Caregiver's Manual* has been a work in progress and will continue to be even after publication of this revised edition. Receiving the recognition of the Florida Council on Aging (FCOA), which awarded the *Manual* the 2013 FCOA Quality Senior Living Award for Senior Vision in Media, has made this effort even more gratifying.

When my editor Brenda and I undertook the Herculean task of preparing this edition of the *Manual*, we knew the content had become even more relevant in the three years since the first edition was published. Those three years saw major developments in the growing need for family caregiver education and support, including new information on a wide range of disabilities and diseases and advancements in the acute care healthcare system that will have long-ranging effects. This new edition is not only an update and enhancement of what we have done previously, but it also underscores the fact that as the number of family caregivers has increased by more than 10 million since 2010, the role of unpaid family caregivers has grown ever more important.

Because of the increasing complexity of care, both clinical and nonclinical, the skill set needed for unpaid family caregiving has never been more formidable. Not in recent memory have our innate human instincts and learned skills been so misaligned with those needed to solve the practical problems encountered by unpaid family caregivers and the broad spectrum of demands placed on them.

While home care provided by paid caregivers is clinical, the tasks performed by informal caregivers are not. Understanding and providing the clinical care required is necessary (e.g., providing correct wound care, ensuring insulin injections are at the proper dosage and given at the proper time, and correctly taking blood pressure). However, as my colleagues and I have monitored the tasks performed by thousands of unpaid family caregivers and paid caregivers in the home over more than twenty-five years, we have found that clinical care comprises only 15 percent of the family caregivers' efforts. The remaining 85 percent of their caregiving time is used for nonclinical care—to do practical problem solving for everything that is not clinical (e.g., addressing legal and insurance issues, arranging medical appointments, providing or arranging for transportation, and resolving family conflict). Moreover, the demands of meeting physical needs typically increase in complexity, as does the challenge of solving day-to-day practical problems such as accessing additional resources.

Thus, the need to prepare today's family caregivers for the inevitable increase in practical problem solving is a given, but we also need to acknowledge that our homes will remain the de facto setting for care. Even now institutional settings are limited and often inadequate in terms of quality of care, and with rapidly increasing demand for care in all settings, finding quality care outside of the home will become increasingly difficult and expensive.

Home is where we are most comfortable and where care is most affordable. There is no "game book" for this, no standardized set of rules, guidelines, and solutions that will meet the diverse care needs of millions of families. The only option available for family caregivers is to have a Plan designed to meet their loved ones' needs and for everyone to be flexible and realize their limitations.

It is becoming very obvious to family caregivers and, at long last, to the public at large and a broad range of decision makers in government and healthcare systems that home-based care provided by unpaid family caregivers is the only viable option for the majority of chronic care in the coming decades. The services provided by community-based organizations are at capacity. Funding from private, state, and federal sources is diminishing. Demands for qualified, paid in-home workers cannot be met. Home-based care is not just *an* option for care—it is a necessity and likely to be the *only* option for care for most families.

Today, many facilities are full or have lengthy waiting lists for admission, while fees for institutional care are rising annually. If placement in a facility is required and can be arranged, the "roof" over the head of the person needing care may change, but the importance of the role of unpaid family caregivers will be unchanged because now they must become active advocates in a non-home setting. As advocates, unpaid family caregivers must act as quality-control agents, following the Plan and monitoring care to ensure their loved ones receive the services they have a right to receive and their dignity and well-being are maintained. Those same unpaid family caregivers need to build new skills and acquire knowledge to effectively work within the bureaucracy that is the long-term care facility system.

Make no mistake: No matter the setting, well into the twenty-first century the backbone and front line of patient care and advocacy will be unpaid family caregivers. Without them, the entire American healthcare system will collapse.

Unpaid family caregiving is constantly morphing. As longevity increases, demographics and family structure change, and cultural and societal adaptations play out, new problems are created even as some problems are solved. Care needs for people of all ages created by chronic illnesses, disabilities, and accidents will not decrease. As the Baby Boomers age, their children, spouses, and significant others will begin to assume the role of family caregiver. Thus, the next few decades will find the United States with upwards of 70 to 80 million unpaid family caregivers.

> **Well into the twenty-first century the backbone and front line of patient care and advocacy will be unpaid family caregivers.**

Typically, the role of unpaid family caregiver is "bestowed" without any formal training, awareness, or support from traditional resources (e.g., doctors, lawyers, financial advisers). New family caregivers who are lucky enough to find available community resources are also likely to find those resources overwhelmed, underfunded, and short of space. This reality will continue to be the norm rather than the exception.

The bulk of America is rural in nature, and local, hands-on family caregiving expertise and resources are limited. Moreover, in reality, because of a lack of preparedness on the part of the "System," this is also the case in urban and suburban areas. Too many family caregivers must depend on the Internet for knowledge. The Internet is an overwhelming "first response" resource but must be utilized with great caution: The bias, accuracy, age of information, and agenda of many websites should be carefully examined before being trusted. The same is true for many individual "experts" who present themselves as reliable sources of unbiased advice. It is far too easy to acquire important-sounding credentials purporting to qualify one as a knowledgeable and competent authority and self-proclaim one's expertise on family caregiving. In particular, the geriatric "Gold Rush" has brought with it clinical and nonclinical charlatans and "snake-oil salesmen" espousing cures and techniques that science has yet to identify, quantify, and prove effective, let alone useful, in treating the diseases and conditions that afflict us most. As always, "let the buyer beware"—unpaid family caregivers should seek to educate themselves before becoming a buyer.

Considering the nature of the caregiving demands in the future, family caregiving should be an area of study in every school's program of instruction, from grade school to post-graduate studies. Family caregivers deserve access to every opportunity to prepare themselves for the challenges they must meet. This manual is a training tool for today's family caregivers and for the family caregivers of the future.

Acknowledgments

This undertaking could not have been possible without the hours, days, and weeks of effort by editor, colleague, and business partner, Brenda K. Bryant. Her years of professional writing and editing were the only reason my caregiver ramblings were shaped into the *Manual*. To her I will be eternally grateful.

Also, I am forever indebted to Sharon Rose, President of Wisdom Production, for her foresight in submitting the *Manual* to the FCOA for award consideration. Without her determination, the recognition of the *Manual* by receiving the award would not have been possible.

I would like to extend a special thanks to the staff of Central Recovery Press for their valiant efforts in editing this new edition of the *Manual*. Brenda and I have long needed other eyes to look, point out our errors and oversights, and help us resolve the usual problems that arise when those who are passionate about content are too close to the words to see. Valerie Killeen and Daniel Kaelin applied their considerable skills at editing, and Deb Tremper her design talents to make the *Manual* even better than it was.

To the thousands of family caregivers with whom I have interacted, I give my undying thanks for the wisdom and insights you have imparted to me over the past twenty-five years and offer my gratitude for your continuing to do so.

To the professionals over the years who have helped me hone my skills and focus my perspective, I must say that without all of you this undertaking never would have been completed. I hope I have contributed my share to our collective pool of knowledge.

I am unendingly thankful for the support and understanding of my wife, Suzette, who led me to my profession as a family caregiver advisor. She constantly supports and endures my laboring in the field that carves out a big portion of our lives—my long hours spent at the computer, in family caregiver support groups, away from home providing individual counseling, and in responding to the ceaseless stream of phone calls and emails from family caregivers worldwide. She is my greatest critic and my staunchest supporter.

Lastly, and equally important, without the undying devotion of Maggie (Bloodhound), Kenzie (Black and Tan Long-Haired Dachshund), Angus (Dappled Red Short-Haired Dachshund), and Mac Jagger (Teddy Bear Pomeranian and *Manual* mascot), this never could have happened.

1.

Today's Family Caregiver

> Past and recent experience has taught us that the family is the primary source of all nonclinical family caregiving. It is also increasingly clear that insurance plans and government programs will never be sufficiently funded, staffed, or motivated to meet all the needs of people who are frail, disabled, or chronically ill, regardless of their ages or the nature of their care.

There is no magic bullet that can make family caregiving easy, but there are practical steps you can take that will make the burden more manageable for you and other caregivers in your family. Therefore, as you work through this manual, you will find explanations of what to do to make family caregiving easier today and going forward.

The American Society on Aging defines a family caregiver as "a person who cares for family—loved ones' elderly or frail; anyone with a physical or mental disability." Other sources refer to "unpaid caregivers" or "informal caregivers." Everyone knows the broadly defined role of the family caregiver, but the role of the individual family caregiver is unique and not so easy to define.

Family: Can it be defined only as a group of people related by blood or marriage? Many people have no blood relatives, no spouse, no siblings, no child—no family in the traditional sense. However, life structures today include partners, significant others, and close friends who are included in the term "loved ones." Many of us depend solely on friends or neighbors to be our real family. The bonds of many kinds of relationships now define what family relationships are, and these newly defined families, along with blood-related families, are today's family caregivers.

Roles of family vary. Caregiving is both a tool and a process. Family caregiving is a tool for providing clinical, rehabilitative, personal, and nonclinical care in home-based locations (home care) to reduce financial burdens on formal healthcare systems. Access to home care provides the clinical care system with a means for people residing in their own homes to receive clinical care, but unpaid family caregivers are the means for providing all social, emotional, practical, and other nonclinical care a person needs to achieve well-being.

Clinical care standards are predictable; what happens in family caregiving is unique and unpredictable. Just as fingerprints differ on each finger and are different from anyone else's, family caregiver "fingerprints" distinguish each care situation from any other. Each family caregiver brings different skills, emotions, attitudes, and problem solving capabilities. Add age, culture, religion, finances, upbringing, family dynamics, and other factors, and it becomes clear that no family caregiving situation could ever be identical. From family to family it may look the same, but no two family caregiving situations are alike, and there is no one formula for creating the perfect caregiving situation.

No two family caregiving situations are alike, and there is no one formula for creating the perfect caregiving situation.

ARE YOU A FAMILY CAREGIVER?

You are a family caregiver if you

- currently provide any level of health, financial, or social assistance in meeting the needs of a family member or friend;

- anticipate being the key person providing assistance or support when someone who is currently managing independently needs assistance or support;
- help someone else by providing care needed by that person's family or friend;
- provide care to someone with special needs who will never be able to fully provide for his or her own independent lifestyle.

You are a **primary caregiver** if you are directly dealing with the care needs of another or are responsible for implementing and guiding the daily care performed by paid or volunteer services.

You are the **alpha caregiver** if you are the one making the final decisions, regardless of who does the daily care. You can be both a primary and an alpha caregiver.

You may be a **local** or a **long-distance caregiver**, depending on the physical distance or practical barriers separating you from your loved one.

Local caregivers live with or close to the person needing care and have personal, day-to-day knowledge of the situation. Local caregivers can visit frequently, if they do not live in the home itself, and directly observe the work of paid caregivers and others who come into the home.

Long-distance caregivers do not live close to the person needing care, or there may be other barriers between the caregiver and the person needing care, such as a contentious family relationship.

Long-distance caregivers face unique challenges because they do not know first-hand and day-to-day what their loved ones are experiencing. They may be alpha caregivers and tasked with making all the decisions, and at the same time, although they rarely see the person needing care, they may be the only primary caregivers available. They must depend on what their loved ones tell them (which may not be reliable), information from agencies they work with over the phone, and paid caregivers or other people they never see face-to-face. When they have the opportunity to visit their loved ones, they sometimes find that information provided is incomplete or inaccurate. Loved ones needing care often hold back critical information. Paid caregivers and agency personnel may not recognize

Regardless of distance, it is always stressful for family caregivers to meet the challenge of ensuring that services are delivered as required.

the degree of change in a loved one's condition or see through the camouflage the person needing care creates to protect his or her dignity and independence. The accuracy of information provided is also dependent on how qualified and professional paid caregivers are; limited skills and interest on the part of paid caregivers can mean that reports on a loved one's well-being are inaccurate and care is inadequate. Dependence on possibly inaccurate information means long-distance caregivers experience a higher degree of anxiety and stress than that experienced by local caregivers who can see for themselves.

Regardless of distance, it is always stressful for family caregivers to meet the challenge of ensuring that services are delivered as required and that care providers offer quality care. For long-distance caregivers, meeting that challenge can be daunting, and that creates a unique caregiver burden.

Family Caregivers Are Jugglers

All family caregivers juggle to find space in busy lives for family caregiving, and the more complex the caregiving situation, the more they have to juggle. For example, many belong to what professionals have labeled the "sandwich generation"; they are caring for aging parents and healthy children at the same time. There are also children who are caregivers, who actually provide hands-on care for siblings, parents, and other relatives at home and struggle to meet the demands of school and simply growing up, in spite of disruptions at home. Family caregivers are of all ages, and because of generational differences in personal, social, work, and familial demands, they have different perceptions of caregiving that influence their approach to caregiving and their expectations of its complexities. They also differ in how caregiving stress affects them.

It *is* possible to effectively coordinate family caregiving with a busy life. Even if you are already caregiving, it is never too late to try new tactics. If you are not caregiving now but see it coming, it is never too early to start getting organized.

The more you learn about what your particular caregiving job will involve, the resources needed to provide care, gaps in resources that require you to adapt your plans, and the kinds of changes that can occur while you provide care, the better able you will be to modify the steps you take so the needs of your loved one are met.

Checklist

DEFINING YOURSELF AS A FAMILY CAREGIVER

What you do for another person who needs care defines you as being a family caregiver. Review the list of common caregiving tasks provided below. Which tasks are you performing now to support someone else's care? Which do you expect to perform in the future? Never? Place a check in the correct column.

CAREGIVING TASK	NOW	FUTURE	NEVER
Call weekly			
Call daily			
Visit several times a year			
Visit weekly			
Visit daily			
Transport my loved one occasionally when other transportation is unavailable			
Transport my loved one regularly to medical appointments, grocery shopping, and vital service points			
Occasionally assist with legal matters			

CAREGIVING TASK	NOW	FUTURE	NEVER
Take the lead in all legal matters			
Occasionally assist with financial matters such as stock purchases and sales			
Take the lead in all financial matters			
Occasionally pay bills and handle banking			
Always pay bills and handle banking			
Occasionally help with household chores			
Perform all household chores			
Arrange for in-home help with chores, shopping, and other daily activities			
My loved one turns to me for all decision-making, planning, and putting things into place			

How many of these tasks do you perform now? _____

How many of these tasks do you expect to perform in the future? _____

If you perform even one of the tasks on this list today, even only occasionally, you are now a nonclinical family caregiver—even if you think you are only getting ready.

From This Point Forward

Many family caregivers may use this manual, and each of them will be caring for different people—mothers, fathers, children, siblings, friends, aunts, uncles, grandparents, neighbors. From this point forward, you generally will not see phrases like "persons needing care" or "loved ones." Rather, you will see names of people or terms like "Mom," "Dad," "Grandpa," "Uncle Ed," "your husband," "your wife," and "your partner." After all, family caregiving is one of the most personal things you can do—it is never neutral.

Keep in mind, also, that while everyone's caregiving situation is unique, quality caregiving shares many of the same characteristics regardless of the setting or the disabilities or chronic illnesses of the people receiving care.

This advertisement could appear in every daily newspaper and on every jobs website.

HELP WANTED

Informal Family Caregiver: Total responsibility for a family member or loved one. Twenty-four hours of work per day. On call seven days per week, fifty-two weeks per year. No pay. No employee benefits. No training. Circumstances change daily—medically, emotionally, and practically. No vacation, no sick days, little to no time off. Job comes with a high stress level and a strong possibility of depression and diminishment or loss of one's social and recreational life.

Must have current knowledge of related legal, financial, practical services, and resources needed to cope with all potential circumstances of caregiving essentials. Extraordinary capability for patience. Must be able to deal with guilt, anger, and resentment. Must be able to find access and use the long-term healthcare system. Must produce practical problem solving solutions on demand. All skills must be learned on the job by accident, luck, or basic intuition. Side benefits: poor health, financial ruin, and loss of self-identity. No terms are negotiable. Apply at: Your Home, Anywhere, USA

2.

Why Planning Counts

Understanding the benefit of planning ahead is sometimes a challenge. Whether you think that one day you may have to be a family caregiver or you are already actively caring for a loved one and feeling the stress of caregiving—planning takes time. Planning will be one more thing on a long list of things to do. However, the time spent planning now can give you more freedom to act later, easing both the burdens and the stresses of family caregiving.

On the following pages you will find three examples of why planning can make a difference, whether you are thinking ahead about caregiving or are in the midst of it.

The stories presented are fictional, but the details are based on real experiences of family caregivers. They represent typical family caregivers: an older man who must work while taking care of his wife who has multiple sclerosis; a young widow who works in a demanding profession and takes care of her two children and now must plan how to care for her grandparents; and a mid-fifties couple who have difficult choices to make when faced with the need to care for their recently paralyzed son.

As you review the stories presented, keep in mind that the function of planning is to provide the family caregiver with peace-of-mind while ensuring the quality of life of the person who needs ongoing support. As you read, consider the following questions, which are written so they represent any family caregiver:

- What kinds of **responsibilities** does the caregiver have to meet?
- What **specific family circumstances** are of concern?
- What **caregiving issues** are of greatest concern in the caregiver's mind?
- Which of those concerns affect **planning and approaches** to the caregiver's tasks?
- What **solutions** are available now?
- What **changes** are likely to occur over time that may alter which solutions work?
- What could the caregiver do now to create more **positive outcomes** down the road?
- In what ways are **your experiences** similar to these caregivers' experiences?

As part of having an effective plan, you need to revisit any plans you develop frequently. The answers to the questions listed above change over the course of time related to both the person being cared for and the caregiver.

Hector and Juana

Hector is a sixty-eight-year-old sales manager for a specialty plastics company, Colco, Inc., located in a major Northeast city. He should have retired at age sixty-five but requested a delay in retirement until he is seventy because he needs the income to support himself and his wife, Juana. Juana, age sixty-seven, has multiple sclerosis (MS), which was diagnosed when she was fifty-five. She has been unable to work since she was fifty-eight because of "brain fog" caused by the MS and was on a modest Social Security disability claim, but when she turned sixty-five enrolled in standard, Medicare Fee-for-Service (FFS).

Because of the economy, Colco has undergone two reorganizations under bankruptcy and Hector's company pension was lost. He too is enrolled in Medicare FFS, has a small Individual Retirement Account (IRA), and has a good benefits plan for legal and dental coverage that the company was able to keep. He and Juana own their small bungalow. He makes a fair living like most people in the area; however, salaries are not that high, even for managers, and Colco hasn't given raises or cost-of-living adjustments since the last bankruptcy in 2007. Hector is feeling the pressure of keeping up sales and dealing with younger sales staff he supervises, all of whom are more than willing to take his place. He feels uneasy about whether Colco will keep their agreement about allowing him to work until age seventy; he is counting on his continued income for at least the next two years and wonders whether Colco's management might find it to the company's advantage to let him go earlier. He also contends with meeting the time demands, emotional demands, and expenses of caregiving, and, at the same time, managing his own health problems—weight and hypertension.

Juana's condition is worsening, and she is now barely able to climb the stairs to the bedrooms in their nearly fifty-year-old bungalow; she needs the help of safety railings on both sides of the stairs. She used to be able to get outside using a cane and was able to get around the house without one, but she now has to use a walker in the house and a wheelchair if they go out. If Juana needs to go to the doctor, Hector typically takes her because the only free medical transport Juana can use is often unavailable. Last week, Hector had to attend a two-day sales meeting in another city. Not only did he have to arrange for someone to stay with Juana while he was gone, but they had to pay for an expensive taxi to take Juana to an important medical appointment. (They have no children and no relatives who live nearby, and this time the neighbors and friends who Hector and Juana have assisted in the past could not or would not provide the needed transportation.)

Hector has reached the point where even the most minor issues upset him, such as Juana preferring more expensive adult diapers while Hector tries to save a few dollars by buying the less expensive ones. He is drinking more, has trouble sleeping, and is in a constant state of anxiety. His doctor tells him repeatedly that he needs to take better care of himself.

Observations

Here are a few observations about Hector's caregiving concerns. Much more could be said. What other observations do you think are important?

Responsibilities: It is critical at this point that Hector keeps his job to continue paying the bills. He has to make sure Juana is cared for now but also needs to prepare for the things she is sure to need to receive care in the future.

Specific family circumstances: There are no family members who can help. Hector is ignoring his own healthcare, creating additional health problems that need to be addressed (use of alcohol, poor diet, high blood pressure). His stress is affecting how he feels when confronted with Juana's requests or demands ("one more thing to do," anger, frustration, and feeling that Juana doesn't understand their need to watch spending).

Caregiving issues: Transportation, the need to prepare their house for Juana's worsening condition or, perhaps, consider selling and moving to a single-story home. Hector must also consider the need to provide increasing amounts of in-home care while he is at work and determine exactly what other resources he might need. For example, Hector may need to seek legal help to qualify his wife for Medicaid. He may need to see if there is a local adult day care Juana could attend and whether it offers door-to-door transportation. He could check with a broker to see what his house is worth and how long the average house on the market takes to sell. If his wife qualifies for Medicaid (which may take care of most of her medical expenses) and he applies for Social Security, he may want to join a no-premium Medicare Advantage program and will need to find out about open enrollment, which plan offers a formulary that matches his prescription needs, whether his physicians are enrolled in the programs he looks at, and the need to provide related resources.

Concerns affecting approaches to tasks: Hector fears retirement, which will be accompanied by greatly reduced income. It is a constant worry that affects his decision-making. Because of increasing stress as he watches Juana's condition deteriorate and her care needs escalate, combined with financial worries, Hector is sliding into depression and becoming less capable of making positive decisions both at home and at work.

Solutions available now: Hector can begin drawing Social Security now, but if he delays until age seventy, he will get the maximum allowed. Because both he and Juana are seniors, there may be services available through government programs in addition to what is covered under Medicare. Hector served in the Coast Guard and may qualify for VA benefits for himself and Juana, and perhaps he can use his legal plan (provided as a company benefit) to speak to an elder law attorney about how Juana can apply for and receive Medicaid to cover increasing expenses and the cost of a nursing home in case she needs one. If a Diversion Program is available under Medicaid, Medicaid may help with providing paid in-home care for a few hours a day. He needs to ask his priest at church this Sunday if they have volunteers who can help out, especially when he has to be away overnight.

Changes that may alter which solutions work: Juana's condition will get worse, and she will need more care. Hector must retire in two years but may lose his job sooner. Hector's health could deteriorate if he doesn't make personal changes, and that, along with his age, will make it harder to find even menial work to supplement post-retirement expenses.

Creating more positive outcomes: Hector needs to find ways to reduce his stress. He knows what the problems are but is stuck on worrying about his job. He sees work as his only solution. Although family caregiving is not a "disease" or, typically, a mental health issue, he might seek the help of a psychologist to talk through his stress and look at alternative ways to make decisions. He may need the help of an elder care/disabled care specialist. He could join a support group for those caring for spouses with chronic illness. He could seek assistance from local, county, and state elder care agencies.

Eleanor

Since starting work just after her marriage, thirty-one-year-old Eleanor has been gradually moving ahead in her position as a financial manager. Her husband, Will, a sergeant in the Army, was killed two years ago while serving in Afghanistan, leaving her alone to take care of their now four-year-old son, Joseph, and two-year-old daughter, Anne, whom he never got to see in person. Will's military life insurance money (which was only $10,000) is dribbling away toward things like home and care upkeep. Her salary is modest, and she gets a small amount of money from the VA to take care of the children. They had no savings when Will died, so things have been tight. Paying the mortgage and paying for childcare is not easy, especially when Joseph has a bout of asthma and his expensive medicines have to be refilled often. Her mother-in-law has offered to take care of the children—to pick them up from day care or stay at Eleanor's house when a child is ill so that Eleanor can work—but Eleanor insists on doing it all herself. So far, she has been making ends meet and has been able to handle things at work and at home without using too many sick leave hours, at least not so many that anyone has seemed to notice.

However, recently she had to begin taking additional time off—her grandparents are having difficulty taking care of day-to-day needs, and she is spending more and more time taking care of things such as tracking and paying their bills. Eleanor was an only child and both of her parents died in a car crash when she was only thirteen. From then on she was raised by her grandparents, who are now in their late seventies and live a few miles from her. Her grandmother, Alice, is still mentally alert but is getting very frail. Eleanor worries about Alice, but it is her grandfather, Joseph Senior, who worries her the most. Lately he has been very forgetful. Eleanor just found out he has been experiencing memory problems for a while, but neither he nor Alice wanted to say anything to her; they do not want to worry her, and Alice is terrified of what may happen if Joseph Senior gets worse.

Observations

Here are a few observations about Eleanor's caregiving concerns. Much more could be said. What other observations do you think are important?

Responsibilities: Child care, elder care, day-to-day demands of work, increasing financial resources for future care, self-care, and the need for her own social interaction.

Specific family circumstances: Eleanor sees herself as the only person who can provide child care. She wants to grow in her profession but is beginning to feel the pressures of both working and raising her children. Her concern for her grandparents, who are the only parents she's really had, have added to her concerns, and she is faced with making even more decisions that will affect how she balances family and work life.

Caregiving issues: Balancing the demands of two distinct types of caregiving (child care versus family caregiving for elders), both of which are likely to increase as Eleanor's children get older and more active socially. Determining the nature and potential severity of her grandfather's memory loss, whether treatment is available, and, if not, what may happen over time.

Concerns affecting approaches to tasks: Growing frustration due to having to put her own plans on hold and unknowns about her children's welfare. She is lonely and wants to add to her own life with some adult companionship. She is using caregiving and child rearing as an excuse not to get out, in spite of her mother-in-law offering to watch the children and help out in other ways.

Solutions available now: See what her church offers in local child care. See if there is a senior center where her grandparents might find social interaction. Does the VA have survivor's benefits in addition to the child-care stipend that Eleanor and her children might be eligible for? Does her workplace have an Employee Assistance Program (EAP) that might help her work out plans for her children or grandparents?

Changes that may alter which solutions work: Further deterioration of either of her grandparent's health, changes in her work circumstances (e.g., a promotion that requires her to spend more time working, slower salary growth due to a perception held by her manager that she is not working as hard as she should), or her son's asthma getting worse and requiring more of her time and money to keep him healthy.

Creating more positive outcomes: Eleanor needs to learn more about her grandparents' financial resources so she knows what she has to work with for their care. If her grandfather does have dementia, she may have to take over management of household expenses and other practical matters he has handled over the years. She also needs to recognize that she does not have to do everything herself. Her mother-in-law, for example, is ready to help with the children at any time. There may also be a local support group for military widows through which she may be able to find emotional and practical support. Also, if her grandfather has dementia, she could join a support group for adult children caring for parents (and grandparents). Eleanor also needs to consider how she is protecting her own children in the event something happens to her.

Ed and Harriet

Ed and Harriet had been very lucky. They ran a successful business together and had been planning for an early retirement (being the same age, both were planning to retire at fifty-five after selling the business), and had a wonderful family. Both of their kids were smart and had a great work ethic. Their daughter, twenty-one-year-old Coral, was working toward a veterinary degree. Their son, nineteen-year-old Ed Junior, was planning on being an engineer. Everything was working out perfectly. Then the accident happened.

Ed Junior had a passion for competitive diving and stayed in the water as much as he could. A few months ago, he and a friend went to Fort Lauderdale to visit Harriet's sister Ellen. They were having a great time, swimming in the ocean, scuba diving, and hanging around the pool at Ellen's housing complex. A couple of days before the boys were scheduled to return home, Ed Junior was playing around on the diving board at the housing complex pool, and he slipped and fell off the high diving board ladder. He fell backward and landed in a way that broke his neck, and he was left paralyzed from the neck down. Everyone hoped the paralysis would be temporary, and he would recover, but it is now clear it is not temporary and nothing further can be done. Ed Junior was transferred from a Florida hospital to take up at least temporary residence in the best extended-care facility near home, but he wants desperately to come home to be with the family.

The bills for insurance deductibles and specialized care are thousands of dollars, and Ed and Harriet's bank accounts are dwindling fast. Their three-story townhouse is in no way ready to accommodate Ed Junior's special needs. Coral is getting ready to begin her advanced degree program, which means more dollars will have to be added to her already high tuition. Ed and Harriet have to keep the business going, which takes both of them.

Observations

Here are a few observations about Ed's and Harriet's caregiving concerns. Much more could be said. What other observations do you think are important?

Responsibilities: Self-care, a father's need to care for his family, a mother's need to care for her children, educational expenses, work demands, fulfilling parents' needs for social engagement, working together as a couple, maintaining a marriage.

Specific family circumstances: Ed and Harriet are concerned about paying for their daughter's education, as well as Ed Junior's care needs and, they hope, his continuing his education. They need to find out if Ed Junior will qualify for Social Security Disability Insurance (SSDI). Posted near the swimming pool diving board were two signs that read, "Dive at your own risk," so Ed Junior's legal rights may be limited.

Ed and Harriet see themselves having to put their plans for early retirement on hold because already their financial resources are being reduced, and they find this frustrating and disappointing. They are concerned about Ed Junior's physical condition, his mental and emotional health, and whether they will be able to meet his expectation of coming home—and how that would affect how they live their own lives.

Caregiving issues: The care that Ed Junior will require if he comes home is unknown, and he is in a short-term care facility. How to figure out what happens next is a challenge. They need the help of a good disability attorney to understand the technicalities of what is available.

Solutions available now: Continue to work together as they always have to solve problems, finding out what would be necessary to bring Ed Junior home and how his physical care needs are to be provided for. They need to take a fresh look at financial resources (including insurance options, especially under the newly enacted Affordable Care Act) to see how to improve their total financial profile in light of current demands. Seek out specialized support from organizations that address spinal cord injury issues (including support groups). Determine whether existing insurance coverage and discretionary savings can be used for uncovered and additional expenses. Their lifelong experience working as a team and good business sense might be used as a foundation for practical problem solving related to family caregiving (e.g., knowing that trained professionals may offer good advice).

Changes that may alter which solutions work: Decline in Ed Junior's physical or mental health, reductions in financial resources, letting personal frustration of their own expectations overcome them, current research in spinal cord injury (e.g., stem cell regeneration) that is showing positive results for treatment and recovery.

Creating more positive outcomes: Was negligence part of Ed Junior's slip and fall from the ladder? If so, they may need to consult a personal injury attorney to consider a lawsuit and a disability attorney about a Special Needs Trust to maintain the proceeds of a possible settlement in order to allow future coverage under SSDI, Medicaid, etc. It might be useful for Ed and Harriet to call a family meeting to let Coral and possibly Ed Junior (if he is mentally and physically strong enough) participate in the decision-making process and allow everyone to share feelings and manage expectations. A review of financial resources could be productive; changes may be necessary in how resources are managed and new options could be put into place (e.g., a different insurance policy, change in how investments are arranged so that some funds are more readily accessed with less loss). A review of legal documents (e.g., wills, healthcare surrogacy documents) may also be helpful.

Money, work, insurance, housing, security, time, care for the healthy and for people needing care, personal expectations and needs, healthcare law, family relationships and dynamics—these and other factors affect how family caregivers feel about caregiving and how they make decisions.

In each of the examples provided in this chapter, the family caregivers had expectations about how their lives would unfold, even though they may not have prepared as much as they should have for their futures or considered that some of life's changes could be so devastating. However, regardless of what plans existed before the need to provide care for a person with a chronic illness or disability arose, the realities of family caregiving always change outcomes for both family caregivers and the people they care for.

None of the caregivers discussed had been trained to be family caregivers. They hadn't thought about being a family caregiver for an adult child or how to prepare to be a family caregiver for someone with severe or chronic health concerns. Their life experiences may have led them to believe they were prepared for anything. If they have experience in planning (for business needs, for example), it is unlikely that they have learned how to transfer planning skills used to meet such needs to planning for caregiving needs. However, family caregiving professionals have found that when faced with the emotional stresses of family caregiving, even the most effective business and medical professionals are too distressed to apply the skills they may demonstrate in a work environment.

> **Family caregivers had expectations about how their lives would unfold, even though they may not have prepared as much as they should have for their futures or considered that some of life's changes could be so devastating.**

Yet, considering the challenges they face, it is clear their success certainly will depend on thinking ahead and learning whatever they can about the caregiving needs that must be met. It also will depend on preparing for the unexpected.

Remember, these are "snapshots" representative of a million different caregiving scenarios. They are included to give you the opportunity to think in terms of planning, instead of just reacting, by recognizing that emotions and inexperience make the task even harder.

The remainder of the Manual can help you become a more prepared, educated caregiver who, in turn, may be better able to face both the expected and the unexpected.

3.

Positive Attitude = Success

To benefit from information, you need to understand why it is needed and how to use it effectively. As a family caregiver, your attitude influences your use of information in a big way.

Whether planning for your own care or the care of someone else, a positive attitude is critical to success. Not believing you can meet the challenges of caregiving is the greatest barrier to effective caregiving. To be an effective family caregiver, you need to put fear and self-doubt aside. Problem solving demands a positive attitude. Believe in yourself as a practical problem solver.

Even effective family caregivers experience doubt or need decision-making reassurance from an uninvolved third party. An objective analysis of a problem and a proposed solution from an understanding, emotionally unengaged third party advisor can be a source of great comfort.

To be an effective family caregiver, you need to put fear and self-doubt aside.

Do Not Overlook Working on Your Attitude

Are you normally a controlling person? You may have to give up some control. Are you afraid of taking control for fear of making mistakes? Learn to overcome fear and take calculated risks. Do you tend to be negative? Work on becoming more positive. Are you depressed and frozen in place? Recognize that being effective depends on a can-do attitude and take steps to overcome your depression.

Being an effective caregiver means accepting help when your can-do attitude is shaky and doubts creep in. Every family caregiver needs support and assistance from others; they need emotional reassurance and guidance for practical problem solving, decision-making, and coping skills.

A positive attitude, combined with practical problem solving, makes a big difference in effective decision-making and attaining positive outcomes.

Good problem solvers are flexible, open to options, and able to try new ideas. They are not discouraged if the first or even second attempt fails.

Are you ready to assess your attitude? Complete the following checklist.

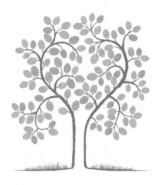

WHAT IS YOUR ATTITUDE ABOUT PRACTICAL PROBLEM SOLVING?

The following ten statements are about attitudes toward problem solving. Which statements do you agree with?

PROBLEM-SOLVING ATTITUDE	AGREE	DISAGREE
1. Having to solve a problem is an opportunity to learn or prove that something can be done.		
2. If I cannot see an immediate solution, I can always look at the problem again and break it down into terms I better understand and can work with.		
3. Problem solving is a process that requires me to define the problem, evaluate possible solutions, and draw conclusions.		
4. There are different sides to every problem and being able to see them makes my analysis more effective.		
5. I do not depend solely on past experience for answers. I expect the unexpected and anticipate the need to look beyond the obvious for solutions.		
6. If conflict surrounds a problem, I am able to recognize and manage the conflict while I find out the facts.		
7. When facts and data are in my hand, I still listen to my intuition.		
8. Once a problem is solved, I continue to anticipate consequences.		
9. When I find what appears to be a permanent solution, I recognize that time and circumstances can create new problems related to the same issue.		
10. When a solution is reached, I get everyone's agreement on and commitment to the solution.		

Do you agree with all ten statements? If you do, you are an exceptional family caregiving problem solver.

Do you disagree with more than three of the ten statements? If so, you may need to reevaluate how you solve problems. What does your disagreement with these statements say about your problem-solving skills? How might your negative attitudes affect your family caregiving? If you had more of a "yes" attitude, what barriers to working with others might be resolved? What can you do to make a positive change in your attitude?

Overcoming Guilt and Resentment

Family caregiving is a very stressful experience because of the high emotional attachment involved. Stress and associated depression can often blind people to their own reactions and emotions they do not recognize. Family caregivers experience depression much more frequently than do people who are not caregiving. Studies conducted by the National Alliance for Caregiving have shown that spouses caring for spouses experience depression six times more often than those not caring for someone, and for people caring for parents or anyone else, it's two times more often.

The greatest roadblocks to effective family caregiving are guilt, anger, and resentment. You already know that having a positive attitude about yourself is essential to you being a good family caregiver and having the best chance for success. Feeling guilty, angry, or resentful can destroy your positive attitude and your chance to succeed.

> **The greatest roadblocks to effective family caregiving are guilt, anger, and resentment.**

Guilt is basically beating yourself up for real or imagined failures in your role of family caregiver. Caregiver guilt can take several forms and family caregivers may experience all of them at once:

- **Remorsefulness/self-reproach:** feeling responsible for wrongdoing, even when what you did worked
- **Sense of inadequacy:** feeling that no matter what you do, you will not do what is needed, and even if you are able to do it, it will not be good enough
- **Self-criticism:** being critical of virtually every task you perform, regardless of whether you performed well or poorly or only believe that you have done so
- **Feeling you acted contrary to personal conscience:** doubting the correctness of your deeds or thoughts

You have a picture of the "Ideal You," an image of what you *should* be, that incorporates all your values and perceptions and represents how you relate to yourself and others. Guilt arises when the day-to-day choices the "Real You" *has* to make, and the choices the "Ideal You" *would* make do not match. As a family caregiver you have to learn that you are not Mother Teresa and Florence Nightingale. There is no perfect caregiving solution, and "OK" is always good enough! You are not the first caregiver and you certainly will not be the last, and not one family caregiver has been, is, or ever will be perfect. So, do not beat yourself up for not being a perfect caregiver.

Note: A parent caring for a special needs child with a chronic or terminal illness has a special kind of guilt associated with the child being denied a "normal" childhood and the parent not being able to be a "normal" parent. This feeling of guilt is made more intense by the slowly growing realization that a lifetime of family caregiving may lie ahead.

Resentment is beating yourself up for what other people did or did not do. Resentment is a lasting, corrosive emotion that leads to feelings of deep and bitter anger or ill will, resulting from real or imagined wrongs. Feeling resentment is a case where "You swallow poison and hope the other person dies."

Resentment comes from unmanaged expectations, that is, when there is a lack of understanding of what may or can happen or promises are made about outcomes that are not met. When treatment or care for Mom does not meet your expectations, resentment can build and become focused anywhere—on hospitals, nurses, home health aides, doctors, insurers, family members, neighbors, or any organization or person who did not do the "more" that would have made Mom's outcome better. Resentment mounts quickly when your social life, friends, and acquaintances dwindle in the face of the demands of long-term caregiving.

Do not beat yourself up for not being a perfect caregiver.

Anger comes from being mad at the System for being so confusing; being mad at friends and neighbors for not understanding what you are going through; and being mad at yourself for not doing "better" when you have no idea what is expected of you. Anger, like resentment, can eat away at your quality of life, well-being, and sanity to the point where the stress it creates is detrimental to your health.

The targets of resentment rarely know about it or couldn't care less. The System is what it is and not what you want it to be. People are who they are and not who you want them to be. Resentment builds when the System and people fail to meet your expectations. Allowed to fester, resentment can distort any situation's reality. Resentment is tough, and lonely!

You are the only player in the game and you cannot win.

Guilt and resentment are self-inflicted and are prevalent in family caregiving. For some insight, consider how professionals define family caregiver: Anyone providing or responsible for unpaid emotional, physical, or practical support and assistance for someone's care needs.

Resentment can grow in a teenage girl because her younger brother is disabled because she has to spend Saturdays taking care of him and cannot go to the movies **The System is what it is and not what you want it to be. People are who they are and not who you want them to be.** with friends, and her needs always seems to get lost in the shuffle—and she may feel guilty for feeling that way. A preteen boy can become angry and act out when he is denied the opportunity to play a sport because Mom cannot share in the after-school carpool because she has to take care of his special needs sister. A son in college can feel guilty because he is away from home and cannot help out with his disabled father, and at the same time, resent that the insurance company will not pay for home care. As an adult caregiver, you can resent family members for not seeing or appreciating you performing the thankless task of managing Uncle Ed's incontinence, personal hygiene, and inappropriate behavior.

Family caregiving is not limited to an age, gender, or particular relationship, nor are anger, guilt, and resentment.

Letting Go

The challenge of providing chronic care is great enough, but when the body is unable to fend off complications the need for care increases and problem-solving solutions that worked before may cease to work. Family caregiving is a dynamic process. Situations can change in a matter of hours. Family caregiving could be described as being dropped into the middle of a foreign country with no knowledge of its language, customs, systems, or structure. Knowing little or nothing, you can barely define your own needs but must engage all of your skills to survive. You must learn to work with a system you know little about in order to care for another human being. On top of that, just when you have begun to understand what to do and how to do it, the problem or the System changes. The survival skills you developed for Problem One are rarely interchangeable for use in solving Problem Two (or Three, Four, or Five).

The prospect of facing daily, problematic sets of ever-varying circumstances with no real wisdom and guidance can cause anyone to become resentful, angry, bitter, and guilt-ridden. These emotions take a deep toll on physical health and well-being and may alienate family, friends, providers, and professionals.

The most broadly accepted family caregiving model is clinically based and depends on acute-care medicine to get people back on their feet, out the hospital door, and back home for long-term, chronic care and lifestyle maintenance (home care). Too often, the patient and the family expect that clinical solutions will resolve all the problems, and medical professionals sometimes foster unreasonable expectations about what medicine can do. However, experience teaches that family caregiving has less to do with clinical issues and more to do with practical problem solving—navigating the clinical and social services bureaucracy (the System), which has little or nothing to do with clinical care. The System is not user-friendly, operates by its own rules, and has a remarkable tendency to minimize input and observations from family caregivers.

The System gives lip service to family-focused delivery but often ignores basic nonclinical needs, such as ascertaining whether an aged stroke victim has anyone to provide care at home, if he or she is sent home on short notice. For example, Dad is a 175-pound stroke victim, and Mom weighs 103 pounds, but no one on the clinical side thinks about the practical issue of how Mom will move Dad out of the bed to the bathroom. This kind of deficiency can cause any family caregiver to feel guilt (at not anticipating such a failure) and resentment (for a System that failed so dramatically to meet the caregiver's expectations).

To let go of resentment toward the System, you must recognize that the System was never designed for long-term care or to address nonclinical matters. To engage effective long-term care, today's patient-focused, follow-the-reimbursement model, must change. Until it does, family caregivers are and will continue to be the backbone and front line for long-term care.

Long-term caregiving is not providing "chicken soup and a good magazine." It is continuous short- and long-term practical problem solving done with little outside support, and its uniqueness makes the problems yours to solve as a family caregiver.

Under such stress, some family caregivers may develop mental health issues and may need individual or group therapy and a mental health professional's help. However, neither caregiving itself nor the emotional distress associated with the caregiving process is a form of mental illness; family caregiving is difficult, but it is not a "disease." Mental health therapy cannot address the lack of understanding of the family caregiving process by the caregiver and the inability of a patient-focused clinical system to respond. Therapists can only act on the associated symptoms.

There are solutions to the emotional stresses family caregivers experience, and both caregivers and professionals who support them can assist in providing those solutions.

1. **Together we must acknowledge that because family caregivers come in every age, size, and relationship, they have unique personal issues.** These issues are both of a practical nature and related to capability, family relationships, and the ability to do the job.

2. **Together we must recognize family caregivers for both the job they do and the personal losses they may suffer.** As reported in 2011 (June, MetLife Study of Caregiving Costs to Working Caregivers), it is estimated that over a work lifetime, an individual family caregiver can lose upwards of $450,000 due to lack of Social Security and retirement contributions, lost income, unpaid leave days, and missed promotions and salary increases. This lack of appreciation of huge personal sacrifices can build deep resentment within a family and in individuals.

Save yourself distress by keeping the following in mind:

- **Remember that no one can be objective in an emotional situation.** Emotion clouds the issues, resulting in confusion and frustration that the family caregiver then internalizes, giving rise to increasing levels of guilt, anger, and resentment. As a family caregiver, learn to acknowledge your emotions and how they affect your thoughts and actions.

- **Accept that as a family caregiver, you need help and support.** Asking family members to help with simple things may stop you from feeling overwhelmed and lessen your feelings of anger, guilt, and resentment.

- **Maintain a sense of balance.** Keep your social contacts, even if you just meet a friend for lunch or a movie; regular social contact is critical for **No one can be objective in an emotional situation.** your own mental health and well-being. No excuses: Having a friend, family member, or paid caregiver stay with Mom for a few hours is perfectly acceptable and necessary.

- **Don't confuse your personal self with your family caregiver role.** Being a caregiver is not who you are; it is what you do.

- **Live life and care for yourself physically and emotionally.** You also need to create or maintain the emotional, social, and economic wherewithal to sustain yourself across the spectrum of personal aging and your own long-term care issues.

- **Access real family caregiver support.** In a family caregiver support group, as opposed to an educational group, you will learn about clinical needs that have to be met, but more importantly you will find practical support leading to a clearer understanding of nonclinical issues and how to be a better practical problem solver. Remember: *85 percent of all family caregiving is nonclinical.* Support groups bring together people with a common role (family caregiving) at different stages and with different illnesses and challenges.

Benefitting from a Support Group

When you join a family caregiver education/support group, you have to know what the group is really about. If the group is not right for you, find another. So, ask questions before joining:

- **What is being discussed and taught?** Is the concentration only on clinical issues (e.g., how to give a bed bath)? Does that kind of information meet your needs? Does the educational content include issues such as how to identify community-based resources, locate additional in-home care, and address your own stresses?

- **Is support brief or ongoing?** Is the program brief (e.g., eight weeks and then you are on your own) or designed to provide ongoing assistance, as your caregiving needs change? Support groups are for the long haul and people come and go. Many of the support groups I have run have been in existence for years, and the variety of experiences make a support group the valuable tool that it is. Many areas of the country have only a few, if any, consistent support groups. Participating using telecommunications tools (e.g., Skype) provided on the Internet can allow you to observe and participate in support groups. Nothing beats being there, but if you cannot attend or a group does not exist near you, watching recordings of actual group meetings is the next best thing.

  If the group is not right for you, find another.

  Avoid pity parties. When new support group participants first join a group, they may start out with a "woe is me" attitude, but an effective group and facilitator can quickly challenge and change that attitude to one of productive interaction focused on more positive outcomes.

- **What does the instructor or facilitator offer? Does he or she have shared experience with the group's caregivers?** The best educational and support groups for caregivers are facilitated by people who, while they may have some clinical knowledge, are trained specifically in nonclinical family caregiving support, practical problem solving, and coping skills. The person may be a paid professional or a volunteer, but he or she should have the training to perform at a professional level specific to addressing the needs of caregivers.

- **Who is in the group?** Are you caring for a parent or your spouse, for a child or a friend? The best support group for you, including those offered in the form of limited-time educational groups, will be one that contains at least a few caregivers who share the same relationship you have with the person they are caring for. Better yet, if you are caring for your spouse, find a group that contains only caregivers caring for spouses; if for a parent, a group for adult children caring for their parents; and so on. However, if you cannot find a group that is dedicated in that way, find a group dedicated to family caregivers in general.

- **After you have participated a few times, did you feel comfortable sharing your emotions and experiences?** A true caregiving support group will provide a safe place for you to express grief, anger, guilt, resentment, and frustration—a place where you can interact with other caregivers who are sensitive to emotional and practical issues because they are also caregivers and where you can receive and provide insight and meaningful responses. The group should treat all things said as confidential, and a judgmental attitude has no place in a support group. Whatever you did or are doing is always subject to constructive interaction, but no one can dictate what is right or wrong for you to do!

The Ultimate Solution

Family caregiving is not intuitive, nor do we have access to a system that has figured out family caregiving any better that we as individuals have. We have no "caregiver gene," and every caregiving situation is unique. Imagine—without the assistance of an experienced family caregiving expert and the support of experienced family caregivers, you and 50 million other caregivers are each reinventing the wheel every day to figure out for yourselves what you need to do. You need more than a list of names and numbers to call or websites to try. You need more than the System saying, essentially, "You figure it out."

What you need is a plan, and building a plan that works for you is what the rest of this manual is about.

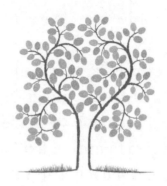

4.

Building a Successful Plan

Imagine being the owner of a small business who wants to expand that business successfully. The owner needs to understand costs, benefits, and options; a wise business owner does necessary research and creates a business plan. It is no different for a family caregiver—a wise family caregiver creates a Nonclinical Care Plan ("Plan").

Making a Plan means preparing for what is happening now and for what may happen in the future, but planning is not always easy. Moreover, most people do not know how to plan or understand the benefits of planning in the context of family caregiving.

An effective plan does the following:

- Defines **purpose.**
- Defines **real and potential problems,** big and small.
- Establishes a framework for **realistic goals.**
- **Communicates** those goals to people who have to make the Plan work.
- Brings together everyone to **better understand** where things are going.
- Helps create **buy-in** and a sense of **responsibility.**

- Develops a clear **focus** to produce more efficient, effective solutions.
- Ensures **effective** resource use.
- Leads to **wiser** decision-making.
- **Measures** success (and failure) so you can make even better choices next time.
- Results in **better outcomes** and **peace-of-mind**.

Keys to Successful Planning

Successful planning depends on cooperation and participation by all parties involved in the caregiving process. Discussions can be held over the phone, via email, or by the exchange of traditional letters. You may wish to have a meeting in which all parties come together (a family meeting). Regardless, the following key issues are likely to be of concern:

- **The guiding purpose of the planning is to maintain the quality-of-life, independence, and dignity of both the family caregiver and the person receiving care.** Each goal and stated outcome of the Plan must support that guiding purpose.
- **Decide how to proceed.** Deciding when to start and who is involved is critical. Delaying starting or avoiding starting altogether assures that nothing will be done before a crisis (or another crisis) arises. Do not think you have unlimited time because nothing critical is happening or it is "early days yet." You cannot determine a turn in the health of your loved one any more than you can be assured you will not have a car accident or a debilitating slip and fall off the "diving board" of life. Family and financial circumstances can change rapidly, and the System is constantly changing, so you need to be ready.

> **Successful planning depends on cooperation and participation by all parties involved.**

- **Planning now is better than planning later or waiting for a crisis to occur.** Planning during a crisis is likely to lead to disaster. The Plan is the key to calmer decision-making and the greater likelihood of success.
- **Do a resource inventory so you can look at available resources** (e.g., people, dollars, time, housing). If you do not understand your resources (financial, emotional, and practical), you cannot make good decisions. You must base every decision on what you have to work with. For example, it

does no good to plan for your disabled sister who is in a wheelchair to live with you if you live on the fifth floor of a building with no elevator. Even front steps can be a barrier. And you have to consider whether the wheelchair can make all the turns in your older home and get through the bathroom door.

- **Identify key choices and issues that will have to be considered in planning.** If you do not have a full understanding of important issues and options for addressing them, it is likely the decisions you make will not work. For example, you need to decide whether your disabled aunt can continue to live at home, but her house is in poor repair and may not be safe, especially when you consider her disability. You must ask: Can the roof be repaired? Can the electricity be rewired? What do you **Develop a shared** do about grab bars and ramps and other things that will **vision as a family.** make the house livable? Is money available from existing resources for repairs and modifications? If not, how can you pay for what has to be done to make the house usable? And, finally, if the changes cannot be paid for, what are the other options? Moving your aunt into a safe and comfortable facility may be the best choice.

- **Be clear about whom the Plan is for and what needs the Plan has to meet.** If goals meet only your personal needs, the needs of the person you are caring for may not be met. If the steps that are to be taken do not meet the situation's needs, the results are not likely to fulfill the desired outcomes. In family caregiving, understanding and addressing real needs is one of the most challenging tasks. For example, everyone, including Dad, needs to agree that rather than keep the family home as an inheritance, it is better to sell Dad's home to pay for nursing care that is essential to his safety and well-being.

- **Develop a shared vision as a family, perhaps during a family meeting (or more than one meeting, if needed).** Families come in all shapes and sizes (and are not necessarily made up of blood relatives). In planning for family caregiving, everyone should have a shared purpose or vision, but reaching that shared vision can be challenging. There may be ten family members who need to agree on whether Dad, who has vascular dementia and is acting out violently against Mom, should be institutionalized. If Mom or one sibling resists moving Dad out, the delay could result in Mom being badly injured. When there is disagreement, at least one family caregiver has to take a leadership role and create a consensus.

- **Consider whether you need the help of a neutral facilitator during a family meeting.** Some family issues are difficult to plan for and quantify. Family members may disagree because of historical differences (e.g., a brother and sister fought as children and are fighting now to see who wins); the nature of personal relationships (e.g., a sister perceives a brother as being egotistical and uncaring about a parent); or because of a personality clash (e.g., Dad's brother, who thinks he is the "boss of everything," versus Dad's protective second wife who does the actual caregiving).

  A neutral party may be able to facilitate the meeting, reframe issues, make objective observations, and get decision makers back on common ground. Your community may offer a number of professionally certified mediators, such as an elder care mediator or a family issues mediator.

- **Prepare a "job description" for the caregiving that has to be done.** Write down the one-time actions (e.g., add grab bars to the bathrooms) and the long-term care tasks (e.g., provide transportation to the doctor every month for the foreseeable future) and consider the kind of help that is most appropriate to perform the needed activity. Everyone needs to know that caregiving is a job and, like all jobs, everybody who "works" in the family has a job description and shares established responsibilities. Share the job description with family members who need to be involved.

- **Pick the leader.** If you are truly on your own as a family caregiver, you may become the alpha caregiver by default, but when there are two or more family members involved in family caregiving, someone has to become the ultimate decision-maker, the alpha caregiver. While the alpha caregiver is the decision-maker, the alpha may not be the primary caregiver providing home support. Perhaps the primary caregiver is not a good decision-maker. Perhaps the person who seems to be acting as the alpha caregiver based on historical interactions at a different time or under different circumstances is no longer the best alpha caregiver for today's circumstances. There may be practical barriers; perhaps the person lives too far away and knows too little about the realities of what is needed to be the one making day-to-day decisions about care. Perhaps you need a "family team" until things are sorted out, and then you may have to choose a more permanent alpha caregiver. Also, perhaps there is self-interest in wanting to be the alpha caregiver, such as controlling Dad's finances to the exclusion of others.

- **Set tasks for everyone.** Large or small, tasks have to be done, and it is important that people know what has to be done, commit to perform their part, and are held accountable. The alpha caregiver can suggest who should do what, and, after discussion and the individuals involved have agreed to share the load, the alpha caregiver should repeat back who has agreed to do what. Your oldest son, away at college, can still provide moral support via phone, e-mail, or text to his chronically ill younger brother. Your daughter, who goes to the same school, can bring home assignments for him and take completed homework to school. These contributions may seem small and insignificant, but not getting homework may make Johnny feel more detached and increase his sense of falling behind. If Mom or Dad are freed up to do more significant things, then the "small" things are equally important as the "large."

- **Agree on key strategies to reach goals.** In family caregiving, this means deciding together how best to use resources to address today's problems and to prepare to meet tomorrow's needs. If your 190-pound brother Ed comes home from Iraq with injuries that leave him facing years of rehabilitation in a wheelchair, can his 103-pound wife Suzy provide physical care, even for a short while? Is home care the right choice and, if so, what equipment is needed and what kind can of paid caregiver assistance is best? What options does the Veteran's Administration offer and for how long? What will happen when Ed and Suzy get older and are less able? Who will care for Ed? What kind of resources will be available to support Suzy after all is said and done?

- **Develop the Plan.** Identify and summarize needs, allocate available resources, identify missing resources, and pinpoint and assign tasks that allow the planners to create and set reasonable timelines.

- **Prioritize.** Put first things first—but the Plan must include future goals, as well as address today's needs. Consider asking the advice of a professional advisor on caregiving to review your efforts and comment on keeping the Plan realistic and workable. Furthermore, an outside professional may have a different perspective on how to be "creative" in dealing with the System and finding local resources.

- **Write it down.** There is an old saying: "If it ain't writ, it ain't real." Even the most well-meaning person can forget spoken agreements. So, write down the Plan and then share the Plan with everyone, including healthcare professionals. With a written Plan in hand, everyone will know what has to be done, when it needs to be done, and who has made the commitment to do it.

- **A written Plan is a tool for ensuring that commitments are met.** Suppose the family members at the family meeting heard your brother Harry say, "I will send $300 a month to help pay for Dad's in-home nursing, and I'll send the check on the fifteenth of the month." After the meeting, no one bothered to write down the individual elements of the Plan. You (the alpha caregiver) and your sister Ellen (the primary caregiver) worked out a monthly budget and included Harry's commitment of $300 to cover costs of hours of paid care. The fifteenth of the month passed and the check from Harry was late. When it did arrive, it was for only $150. Because you are the alpha caregiver, you called Harry up and said, "Thanks for the check Harry, but we were wondering when the remaining $150 will get here? Oh, by the way, Ellen really needs you to send the check by the fifteenth as you agreed." Harry responded, "Hey, I didn't agree to send $300 a month every month! I said maybe $150 every couple of months, *if* I can." Without the written Plan in hand to review and refresh his memory about his commitment, Harry's contribution not only shrank, it also became an "if."

- **Review the Plan frequently and revise it as often as necessary.** Human beings are prone to forget about small and large commitments and time frames in which we have committed to do something. Reviewing the Plan at least monthly (and whenever something happens that may require you to make a change) is a must.

Nothing is certain in life; family caregiving is no exception. Every day and every hour of caregiving is different and can bring a change. Tasks included in the Plan when it was written last month can change this month, or two days after the Plan was written, for that matter. For example, your fifty-year-old mother, who lives alone with minimal supervision, has mental health issues severe enough that you are now her legal guardian. Suddenly, she begins to demonstrate delusional behavior. She renewed her prescriptions when she last went to the psychiatrist, but you checked and the dosages were the same (dosage changes can cause side effects in any treatment regime). When the doctor sees Mom, he decides that her behavior is not a result of medication issues, but that her condition has deteriorated. She can no longer be left alone at any time. So, you

> **The only constant in family caregiving is change. Recognize it and be prepared for it.**

have to figure out the options, reallocate tasks and resources, and revise the Plan, yet again.

One of the things family caregiving guarantees is that nothing stays the same. As soon as things seem to be running smoothly and on course, an event or circumstance occurs that flips things upside down. The only constant in family caregiving is change. Recognize it and be prepared for it.

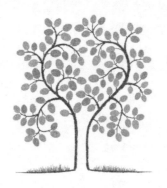

5.

Why Document?

Whether you have limited resources (a single paycheck) or extensive resources (healthy retirement and investment plans, property, etc.), up-to-date and correctly prepared financial, legal, and healthcare documentation makes it easier to make decisions and can protect everybody's rights. Even if you are not in the throes of developing a Caregiving Plan for a loved one, having access to up-to-date information is important—for everyone, regardless of their age, health, or anticipated needs. Having accurate, complete information is vital for developing a functional Plan.

Let's suppose Mom, who is a widow, is beginning to feel frail, and she wants you and your sibling to work together to plan ahead, just to be prepared in case something should happen. If you have gathered together essential information about her situation, you should be able to answer yes to the following five questions:

1. Have the two of you recently reviewed Mom's **financial and legal documentation** to identify any gaps in financial plans (records, asset protection plans, insurance) and legal documentation (wills, deeds, powers of attorney, advanced healthcare directives, and living wills)?

2. Do **legal documents** include those that have been recently revised to ensure healthcare information, coverage, and preferences (and a Caregiving Plan)? Are they up-to-date in terms of changes in local, state, and federal laws and rules and can they be used without difficulty (including medical history, healthcare provider lists, legal documents covering healthcare surrogacy instructions and designations)?

3. Is all this critical information **assembled in one place**?

4. **Is it accessible**? Information locked in an inaccessible safety deposit box or Dad's home safe is as good as no information at all.

5. Is the information **organized** so that needed answers can be found quickly, not only by you and Mom but by someone who might have to step up in a crisis?

There is also a sixth, and final, question you should be able to answer yes to:

6. Have similar legal documents been prepared and information gathered **for all family members of legal age**? (Remember Ed Junior? He did not plan to fall from the diving board, but that fall was a life-changing event at age twenty-four. How different would things have been if documentation and a Plan had been in place?)

When you are preparing a Caregiving Plan, even the smallest details may one day be important.

Were you able to answer yes to all six questions? If you were, well done, but do not forget to review the information and update as needed. If you were not, everyone has wo rk to do. The sections that follow will assist you in your preparation.

What Can You Learn?

You may know a great deal about the person you care for, or you may know very little. When you are preparing a Caregiving Plan, even the smallest details may one day be important.

Regardless of where someone is in the spectrum of care process—even if there is no immediate concern—by developing a complete picture of a person's background and resources, you can determine next steps. The next step may simply be planning for savings and investments, or it may be reorganizing to ensure that an effective

Caregiving Plan can be put into place. You need to consider the same questions regardless of where someone is in the care process.

- **Are plans in place for long-term care?** Are you managing assets and income for maximum coverage and protection? Have you considered legal and financial incapacity?

- **Is care likely to be needed in the future,** considering current health conditions and family conditions? If the last three generations of women on Mom's side of the family had Alzheimer's disease, it may be reasonable to consider that Mom or her daughters may get it, in spite of having no current symptoms.

- **What preferences does the person have** for where (location) and from whom to receive such care?

- Can **the family and social network** provide that care?

- Can **valuable information** be gathered now that will assist when the care need arises?

- Are **local community services and programs** available that can be accessed for needed care? What is the likelihood that they will remain or be funded going forward? Changes in health law and funding change resources.

- **Before care is needed**, what services should you familiarize yourself with (special needs child care, assisted living, adult day care, visiting nurses, VA hospital locations, autism specialists)?

- **What steps will maximize independence**, dignity, and quality-of-life for the family caregiver and the person being cared for?

Even a young person can begin thinking about these questions. It is never too early to plan.

Does Everyone Need Legal Documents?

Absolutely! To ensure effective family caregiving, essential documents should be in place for every family member. Being young and "invincible" does not guarantee protection against illness or accident any more than age guarantees it. Everyone must prepare for the unexpected by putting healthcare documents in place, especially when the relationship is a domestic partnership (unmarried or with significant others). Without proper documents the law will not permit someone to share in personal information nor can that person participate in essential decision-making.

Durable Powers of Attorney are essential, and the legal rights of the people in every relationship need to be formally in place. No matter what the relationship may be, or how long it has been in place, or what has been said, even in front of witnesses—without valid formal documentation there is little that can be readily done. This is also true for adult children acting on behalf of parents and grandparents or siblings acting for siblings. Without legal documents, you have no greater rights than a total stranger.

While a doctor or healthcare provider may accommodate you with basic information in an emergency situation, the rest of the System may not. Something as simple as accessing prescription information at a pharmacy may not be allowed. You may have a great relationship with your aunt's primary care doctor who may cooperate in keeping you informed, but what happens if your aunt falls ill and her doctor is on a vacation or a business trip?

Having access is also important if you have to gather needed information for tax purposes at the end of the year on unreimbursed prescription expenses, or write checks to pay your aunt's bills, or access her safety deposit box. The ability to sign her into a nursing home or assisted living facility will be severely limited without a Durable Powers of Attorney with Medical Authority, and you may wind up being financially responsible without the legal protections that are built into such documents. Contracts and documents for care and services need to be carefully reviewed. If you are unsure about the contract, consult a professional.

Get It Organized—Make It Handy!

Being organized and ready now saves time and worry later. Remember: Anyone at any age can be "hit by a bus" and be just as incapacitated as someone with a chronic or terminal illness, such as multiple sclerosis or Alzheimer's disease.

Information on who makes healthcare decisions when Mom cannot make them should be in the charts of her primary healthcare provider and all her specialists.

The documents need to be up-to-date, state-specific, and available to designated family members or friends when the need arises.

Copies of legal documents should be kept by the lawyer who prepared them and provided to any individual named in the documents as having decision-making authority. States and financial institutions may require documents that bear original signatures be presented, posing special concerns for long-distance family caregivers. *Know what is needed.* Do not assume photocopies and faxes will always suffice; many institutions only accept original documents.

Designated family members should know what steps need to be taken and when. They should have copies of documents in which they are named as being legally empowered to act.

Copies of legal and financial documentation need to be readily available. Because banks are not always open and emergencies can occur at anytime, safety deposit boxes may not be the best places to keep originals of critical documents. If you do not know the combination to your brother's wall safe, having documents in it can be equally problematic in a crisis.

The importance of advanced organization cannot be overemphasized, especially in regard to healthcare. Having a well-organized set of legal and patient history documents in hand when visiting a new (or an old) healthcare provider and providing copies to physicians, hospitals, and so forth to be included in a patient's file can help you establish healthcare surrogacy rights, patient preferences, and legal status. Providing healthcare records, for example, as related to allergies, can help prevent inappropriate treatment and accidents due to ignorance.

In case of emergency, healthcare information may also be written out and attached to Dad's refrigerator door. Many emergency medical technicians (EMTs) are trained to look for it there, or if Dad needs to and he is able, he can tell someone where to look.

Time is precious in an emergency, and readily available key documentation makes the job easier and a positive outcome more likely. The illustration on the following page is a sample of just such a form.

Emergency Notification Information Summary			
Person's Name			
Closest Major Cross Streets			
Phone Number			
Primary Physician			
Primary Physician's Phone Number			
Preferred Hospital			
Hospital Phone Number			
Assistive Devices Used, Dentures, Contacts, Eyeglasses?			
Language Spoken			
Medical Conditions (including Dementia) This Person Has			
Allergies This Person Has			
Medications This Person Takes	Name	Dosage	Frequency
Emergency Contact	Name: _____		
	Cell Phone: _____		
	Other Phone: _____		

MAKE COPIES OF THIS PAGE. POST IT ON THE REFRIGERATOR.
UPDATE IT AS NECESSARY.

Tips for Efficiently Organizing Information

- Place original documents and other written records in **folders labeled by category**.

- If you are gathering information for more than one person, have a **separate set of folders with all categories for each person**. Remember that even though you may consider something a joint asset, if only one name is on a deed or similar document, that asset is solely owned by that person.

- As you go along, **scan original documents to preserve a record** should anything happen to the original documents. Once you have a complete file in digital form, you can copy that file and put one copy away for safety, keep one copy on your computer, and share the information as needed with others.

- Keep health-related documents handy by scanning them and then transferring them to **flash drives,** from which they can be downloaded when needed. Some drives can be attached to a key chain, and some come in the form of credit-card sized flat drive that can be kept in a wallet or purse. If original signatures are required on documents, the fact that a copy is available until the original can be shown may be useful in convincing someone that you or a designated party may make decisions for another person. Be sure to take precautions to protect the information on the drive—block out Social Security Numbers and insurance plan numbers when you can, use document passwords, and only store essential documents.

- If you know how to use a computerized spreadsheet tool, such as Microsoft Excel, it might be useful to **set up a spreadsheet** in which you can enter and summarize the dollar value of those categories as needed.

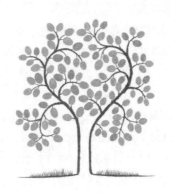

6.

Critical Information—The Lists

Gathering information may require a lot of patience and time, but it is critical to the planning process. The list provided below incorporates a comprehensive body of information that can form a firm foundation for planning to meet today's immediate needs and identifying needs and options over the long term, as well as for rapidly adapting plans when crises or major changes in needs occur in the short term. You can use the "Family Caregiver Questionnaire" provided in the back of the *Manual* or any other means you feel comfortable with to record the information you gather.

Some points to keep in mind:

- **Do not be intimidated by the list's length.** It is only a guide developed to assist in gathering as much vital information as possible.
- **The list is broken into two sections:** 1) For the family caregiver and 2) For the person needing care now or who may need care later. Categories of information range from health to family to legal and financial.
- **Some items, even entire sections, may not be relevant in the Plan you are developing today,** but do keep in mind that they may be important

tomorrow. As already noted, the more you know the better, even if you don't consider it useful now.

- **The information may be readily available and easy to work with or hard to find** (or even not exist) and a source of problems (e.g., a will that is thirty years old names a divorced spouse as primary beneficiary).

- **Not all items in the list will apply to every person,** but this list should be reviewed and information provided for each person who now requires care and for people who may require care in the near future. The fact is that you should gather a basic set of information for everyone you consider a member of the family, whether related by blood or not. People's needs change and basic information can be monitored and modified as time goes on (annually, biannually, or after a life-changing incident) so that everyone is prepared to make long-term plans when needed and respond quickly when crises occur.

- **There may be unique information about you or a loved one that is not covered in this list,** but that may be relevant to any Plan you make. Be sure to include that unique information in your documentation.

- **Missing information, such as wills and surrogacy documents, are critical gaps.** Not being able to find some information, such as the year a person graduated from high school, will not create major issues, but the lack of a valid birth certificate may.

- **Being patient is crucial.** If you cannot locate all information about a specific item, list what you do know and continue to investigate. Consider who may have the information or know where to find it. Do not forget online databases for birth and death records, family trees, and social media sites to identify people with prior work and personal relationships who may be able to fill in the blanks.

Some people have financial, legal, and health records that are legible, straightforward, and comprehensive. They may have a savings account, wages, health insurance, life insurance, and a will. Other people's lives are crowded with information—investments, real estate, trusts, multiple bank accounts, and so forth. People differ in how they store and recall information, regardless of its nature. You and your wife may be organized and have meticulous records. However, your wife's seventy-year-old uncle, David, may have a desk crowded with bits of paper, boxes under the bed and in the attic, and safety deposit boxes at five different banks crowded with information, stock certificates, and on and on, and no one, not even Uncle David, knows which documents are accurate and up-to-date, let alone what information is in which box.

Regardless of the circumstances and the challenges, getting an accurate picture of what resources are available in developing a Caregiving Plan for a loved one is absolutely necessary. The future of people who may have to depend on those same resources later and how to ensure they are protected should also be considered. More problems will arise if every dollar from all resources is used to care for Uncle David, leaving nothing for his sixty-two-year-old wife, Helen, to live on after he has died.

Some of what you need to know, such as language spoken and educational history, has to do with the person's cultural background. This kind of information is important because it may influence the person's attitudes and choices. The more you know about the person you are caring for (or people know about you if you need care), the better you will understand what that person may want and why he or she acts a certain way. The more you know, the easier it will be to identify the kind of care needed and the resources available to meet those care needs today and tomorrow.

A word of caution: Some individuals may withhold information because they think that if they openly share information on their ethnic, religious, cultural, or socioeconomic background or lifestyle a healthcare provider or some other "authority" will either react with prejudice toward them or use the information in a negative way (e.g., deny care). No one can say that will not happen because no one can predict when and where any of us will encounter a person who is prejudiced. However, responsible care providers who know about ethnic and cultural background, religious preferences, preferred language, and other lifestyle issues can use that information to create opportunities to provide better care, because they can anticipate difficulties in communicating and be aware that there may be customs, traits, and idiosyncrasies that will come into play.

The Family Caregiver Questionnaire, a convenient form to use when documenting information, is provided at the end of the *Manual*. You can also obtain additional copies of The Family Caregiver Questionnaire from the Family Caregiver Advocacy Group by visiting www.caregiverreality.com and selecting the "Shop" page option.

The Caregiver's List

Prepare a summary of the following information about yourself. Some of what you list, contact information for example, can be provided to other family members who help with caregiving, in-home paid caregivers, medical professionals, or others as needed. You will use other information, such as your personal goals, in planning how you will work as a family caregiver.

A. **Your current contact information** (address, cell phone, home phone, work phone, primary email, other contact information).

B. **Your marital status** (single, married, separated, divorced, domestic partnership).

C. **Relationship to the person being cared for**
   1. Type of relationship.
   2. Do you live with this person? If not, where do you live?
   3. Does this make you a local or long distance caregiver?

D. **Your family caregiver responsibilities**
   1. Are you a decision-maker, a hands-on caregiver, or both?
   2. If you are currently providing care, how long have you been providing care?
   3. What is your expectation as to how long you may be required to continue to provide care for this person?
   4. Who assists you? List name, relationship to you, relationship to the person being cared for, contact information (and be clear in stating where they live because they should have different tasks based on if they live locally or at a distance) and their occupation.
   5. What tasks do you perform now?

6. What tasks do you expect to perform in the near term and in the future?

7. How would you describe your emotional state? Attitude? Stress level? (If you have not done so already, find the "Problem-Solving Attitude" and "Caregiver Stress" checklists in the *Manual* and complete them.)

E. **Goals**

1. List your current goals as a family caregiver.

2. List your current goals for your personal well-being.

3. List what you feel are your physical, financial, and emotional limitations in providing care for your loved one.

The List for the Person Needing Care Now or in the Future

The information in this list forms the foundation for care planning by clarifying issues. As you work through this, you will identify gaps that have to be filled (e.g., necessary legal documents for the person are missing, there is no list of medications and it has to be prepared).

You should also prepare a list like this for yourself, other legal-age family members, and others you may be providing care for in the future; it is never too early to plan. (You can make additional copies of the Family Caregiver Questionnaire at the back of the Manual to use for each person.)

PERSONAL DATA
Section I. Key Information

A. **Current photo in color:** The photo should be full face and the face image should be at least 2½ inches high so features can be clearly seen. Also, keep *current* full-face and full-height photos on your cell phone and computer that can be used to identify your loved one should he or she wander off, drive off, or be missing. A twenty-year-old photo from the last cruise Uncle Fred took is not going to be helpful.

B. **Descriptive information:** Birthdate, age, height, weight, blood type, birthmarks/scars, tattoos, skin color. The photo and descriptive information is vital in some circumstances. For example, if more than one person of the same gender and general description lives in the home or if someone has dementia and wanders away—knowing what the person looks like today will help searchers know when the wanderer has been located.

C. **Identification document(s):** Driver's license or state approved identification card, passport, residence status document with the passport, any other forms of legal identification available. (Note: Person being cared for should always carry identification documents and emergency contact information.).

D. **Insurance and benefit numbers:** Including healthcare insurance (name of provider, individual and/or group policy numbers, contact number for company), Social Security number, Medicare number, Medicaid number, Veterans ID number.

E. **Language:** Primary language spoken and level of usage. If the person being cared for speaks a language other than the primary language spoken in the country where he or she is living, it is important to make it clear to ensure healthcare providers, emergency workers, and others the person has to interact with know whether a translator is needed or if special care has to be taken when communicating. For example, your grandmother may have been born in Poland and speaks only a little English, or she may speak English fluently; a doctor needs to know which. Also, depending on medical circumstances, a person may revert to speaking his or her native language in a crisis.

F. **Marital status:** Single, married and living with spouse, married and not living with spouse, divorced, living with significant other, etc.

G. **List of the following items:**
   1. Phone numbers for the person needing care and a person to be contacted in an emergency: cell, home, business.
   2. Email addresses: personal and business.
   3. Name of spouse/significant other (or emergency contact and his or her relationship to the person needing care if this does not apply).

4. Address of spouse/significant other (or emergency contact) if different from that of person needing care.

5. Healthcare provider list (names, phone numbers) including primary physician, specialists, primary pharmacy and medications it provides.

 TIP: The Medication List: It is essential that you prepare and regularly update a list that includes both prescription and over-the-counter medications that can be provided to all medical professionals to avoid over-prescribing and damaging medication interactions. It is very important to keep the updated list handy so that it can be found easily when it is needed in emergencies.

6. Type and locations of critical legal documents: name of designated power of attorney with contact phone numbers, location of advanced directives, name and contact phone numbers for designated healthcare surrogate if this person is not also the designated power of attorney.

Section II. Health Insurance

A person may have several types of insurance, depending on age and circumstances, including one or more of the following: individual and group healthcare policies provided by employer or through private purchase, Medicare (FFS), Medicare supplement, Medicare Plan D (drug coverage), Medicare Advantage Plan, Veterans Benefits, Medicaid, major medical, long-term care insurance, dental, short- and long-term disability, accident, cash for healthcare expenses. List and describe all.

A. Provider name

B. Policy holder ID number

C. Type of insurance

D. Fees for service(s)

E. Claims support number

F. Which services require preapproval

Section III. Military Service History and Veterans Benefits

A. Veteran's serial number

B. Branch of service

C. Highest rank attained

D. Enlistment date

E. Discharge date

F. Place discharged (base, city, state)

G. Served during time of combat (yes/no); if yes, where and when?

H. Wounded in combat? If yes, describe.

Section IV. Medical Care

A. Manages own medicines, makes and keeps doctor appointments or, if not, who does this?

B. Does the person get regular preventive care for health and dental conditions? If not, why not?

C. Last Physical: date, done by whom, where given, contact information.

D. All tests done (e.g., blood, scans, x-rays, EKG, urinalysis, cognitive function tests).

E. Results/major findings found where?

F. Recommended post-exam care or follow-up (date, time, location).

G. In the past twelve months, has this person experienced one or more health-related incidents, such as a serious fall, diagnosis of a new chronic condition, major change for the worse or better in an existing chronic condition? If so, describe the event and the changes that it has caused.

H. How often does the person visit physicians or healthcare providers? Why? Provide name of provider, frequency of visit, and reason.

Section V. Capabilities and Other Issues

A. **Capabilities**

In this section, indicate whether the person performs the following tasks always, sometimes, or never.

- Does own shopping for groceries and other items (including clothes)
- Prepares own meals
- Handles personal hygiene needs (e.g., bathing, hair care, dressing)
- Manages own finances (e.g., pays bills, balances checkbook)
- Does housekeeping chores and does/does not require assistance
- Drives or otherwise manages personal transportation needs; has current license tags, driver's license, and vehicle insurance
- Has chronic conditions: List all (e.g., high blood pressure, arthritis, diabetes)
- Uses assistive devices (e.g., wheelchair, walker, cane, hearing aid, glasses, dentures, etc.)
- Is occasionally confused or forgetful
- Seems moody or depressed
- Takes good care of him/herself (e.g., maintains good hygiene, personal appearance)
- Is beginning to rely more on others

B. **Other Issues**: List all that apply.

- Currently smokes (Describe effects)
- Smoked in the past (Describe effects; indicate when quit)
- Has trouble hearing (Describe effects)
- Uses a hearing aid (Describe effects)
- Has good vision
- Has impaired vision: list type of impairment (e.g., glaucoma, macular degeneration, cataracts) and describe effects
- Wears contacts or glasses (Nearsighted? Farsighted? Other?)
- Had corrective eye surgery (Describe, including when done and after-effects)
- Wears dentures (How old are they? Do they fit well?)

- Has artificial limb or other prosthesis (Describe)
- Has insulin pump (Date inserted)
- Has pacemaker (Date inserted)
- Has pain pump (Date inserted)
- Being tube fed (For how long? Is there a central line?)
- Needs oxygen (How received, home or portable pump? Other method?)
- Currently in dialysis (When begun, frequency, name of provider and location(s) in which provided, and how does the person get there?)
- Weight (Ever diagnosed as overweight? Underweight? Was reason known?)
- Recently gained/lost weight (How much and is reason known?)
- Feels fatigue/weakness (Is reason known?)

Section VI. Family Caregiver Responsibilities

A person needing care may also be a family caregiver. If so, you may have to plan for alternative family caregivers if that person becomes unable to continue providing care.

A. Relationship to the person(s) being cared for

B. Name of person(s)

C. Is person being cared for an adult or a child?

D. Why does the person need care (physical or mental healthcare issue, seriousness)?

E. How long has the person been providing care?

F. Description of the family caregiving situation (e.g., type of care, location of care)

G. Assisted by (name, contact information, relationship to primary caregiver and person or persons being cared for)

H. Does the person express concerns over his or her ability to be a family caregiver? Describe.

Section VII. Lifestyle Information

A. **Education background and literacy level**

   1. Where educated (elementary, junior high, high school, college, graduate school, technical school; years attended, graduation dates, major[s], degrees earned)

   2. Classes currently enrolled in

B. **Work History**

   1. Retired? When?

   2. Current or last occupation (title, description including hours worked, years worked, perception of stress in occupation (high, moderate, low), level of activity (active, semi-active, inactive), hazardous occupation (e.g., mining, exposure to asbestos)

   3. One or two previous occupations with same information

   4. Is the person currently volunteering his or her time? (If so, where, how many hours, and type of service?)

C. **Children (if any)**

   1. Name

   2. Sex

   3. Age

   4. Deceased (when, cause of death)

   5. If living, whether lives in same household or city and state of residence

   6. Racial heritage (especially relevant to adopted children and "second" families because it may influence decision-making)

   7. Does the child help in caregiving? If so, for whom and what does the child do, and how often?

D. **Living Situation**

   1. Living arrangements: owns home (single family, apartment/condominium), rents (single family, apartment/condominium, duplex, or multiplex), planned community, special needs apartment or house, assisted living facility (single or shared space), nursing home (single or shared space), life community (different levels of care from independent to nursing care provided)

2. Lives alone

3. Lives with other people: name(s), relationships, contact numbers (cell, home, work), email addresses

E. **Type of Housing**

   Note: A Safety Checklist is provided on page 134 of the *Manual* that you can use to evaluate the home in detail and that can provide you with up-to-date information for this section.

   1. Type of residence (single family, townhouse, duplex, multiplex, apartment building, independent/assisted living, other)

   2. Number of stories

   3. Steps to get inside

   4. Floor if living in apartment

   5. Elevator or stairs between floors

   6. Number of access doors to home or apartment and location (type of locks)

   7. Location of bedrooms/baths (On which floors, if multistory?)

   8. Room for live-in help (private room and bath, for example)

   9. General condition of residence and grounds

   10. Maintenance contracts (grounds, appliances, and/or systems, such as plumbing) and what is covered for what time period (renewal date)

   11. Adaptations for disabled/frail

       a. Existing ramps that meet code, elevators or lift chairs in residence, grab bars and similar assistive devices, paddle handles on doors, etc.

       b. Modifications needed to accommodate disability/frailty

   12. Repairs or maintenance needed and what kind specifically (roof repair, roof replacement, grounds, building outside, building inside), repair or replacement/remodel (bathroom, plumbing, electrical, furnace, air conditioning, kitchen, appliances, lighting both interior and exterior, stairs inside and out, windows and doors, exterior and interior walls), any other areas of concern

F. **Transportation**

    1. Drives? State and renewal date of driver's license

    2. Has own car? Condition of car, any special equipment (such as adaptation for disability)

    3. Handicapped placard or plates (permanent or temporary)?

    4. If he or she does not drive, type of transportation used (e.g., public, family member, bus provided by city/county)

    5. Public transportation provided convenient to residence? Type?

    6. Is disabled, medical, or senior transportation available?

    7. Does person use public transportation? Is a bus/rail pass used and when does it expire?

G. **Nutrition and Dining Habits**

    1. Dietary restriction (Describe.)

    2. Favorite foods (Are these off limits because of dietary restrictions?)

    3. Prepares own meals at home (If not, how are meals provided and name of person or service that provides the meals.)

    4. At home, dines with someone or alone?

    5. Eats out (Frequency? Where? restaurant, congregate meal site for seniors and its location, other person's home)

    6. Average cost per eat-out meal, if pays personally

H. **Physical Activity**

    1. Type (none, walking, biking, swimming, jogging, aerobics, strength exercises, yard work/mowing lawn, household chores, other)

    2. Gets thirty minutes or more of exercise appropriate for age and condition three or more times a week

    3. Uses a gym (goes to a gym or has equipment and uses it at home)

I. **Social, Cultural, Other Activities**
Describe activities currently engages in (type, locations, frequency)

    1. Interests (music, art, history, other)

    2. Hobbies

    3. Organizations and social groups belongs to and attends

    4. Religious activities

    5. Other

J. **Pets**

    1. Type, names, ages

    2. Can person properly care for pets under present circumstances?

    3. Cost of food and care

    4. Pet sitters who can be contacted for emergency pet care

    5. Veterinarian contact information and after hours pet hospital

Section VIII: Medical History

A. **Family Medical History**

Note: A thorough family medical history can aid medical professionals in tracing genetic and lifestyle patterns that may affect or have affected a person's health—important in diagnosing illnesses.

    1. List information for the following individuals, if possible: father, mother, grandfather and grandmother on father's side, grandfather and grandmother on mother's side, mother's and father's siblings (person's aunts and uncles), person's siblings.

    2. Indicate year of birth and age, if living; year of death and age, if deceased; current health conditions, if living; cause of death, if deceased; major conditions such as heart disease, diabetes, or dementia.

    3. Does this record reveal information that indicates conditions on either side of the person's blood-related family that appear to be a pattern of genetic/inheritable diseases? If so, describe them.

B. **Allergies**

    1. All medications (including vitamins) that are **not to be taken**.

        a. Prescription medications (by brand name or by generic name if taken as generic)

        b. Over-the-counter (OTC)

        c. Homeopathic

        d. Herbal

e.   Alternative

2.   List all allergies to foods, cosmetics, detergents, etc., and describe the person's reactions.

3.   Has the person been tested to verify that what appear to be symptoms of allergies are indeed allergy symptoms and to determine hidden allergies? How long ago? (Some "allergy" symptoms are really signs of other illnesses. Some allergies are hidden until first-time exposure or exposure levels reach a critical level. Some allergies disappear over time.)

C. **Dementia**

If you think the person has a memory issue or dementia but a diagnosis has not been made, it is recommended that a qualified neurologist evaluate the person to confirm a diagnosis before any medication is given. The type of dementia will determine the kind of medication or other treatment provided. This evaluation may include a general physical examination, psychometric testing, and brain scans to determine other possible conditions; a review of medications and recent changes in medications that might induce memory change; and cognitive function tests, neurological exams, and other "best practice" evaluations to determine dementia.

If the person has been diagnosed as having a form of dementia, please provide information listed below.

1.   List type of dementia and stage of disease when tested

2.   When diagnosed

3.   Behavior or other issues shown by person; it is helpful to keep a daily record showing time and type of issues that appear, such as late afternoon fatigue and irritability (called "sundowning"), hallucinations, fear, and paranoia

4.   Medication name, dosage, frequency dosage is taken, and whether person takes the drug without assistance or the drug is administered by others

5.   Have you noticed a progression of symptoms in the last twelve months (again, a daily record of behavior can be helpful in evaluating this)?

D. **Additional Conditions and Medications Taken**
Include prescriptions, over-the-counter, homeopathic, alternative, herbal, vitamins.

1. List the condition being medicated, medication name, dosage, frequency dosage is taken, whether person takes the drug without assistance, or if the drug administered by others.

2. Be sure to include sleeplessness, arthritis, pain, high blood pressure, high cholesterol, fluid/edema, cardiac conditions (all), diabetes (list type), depression, stress, osteoporosis, thyroid condition (type), stomach condition (type), eye condition (type), vitamin deficiency, preventive vitamin therapy, dementia (list type, such as Alzheimer's disease, vascular, frontal temporal lobe).

3. Even if a person has a condition that is under control through the use of medications, list the condition and say it is under control (e.g., if a person takes medication to keep blood pressure down and the medication works, the person still has high blood pressure).

E. **Vaccinations**
List date first given, any reactions, most recent booster, any reactions to booster.

1. Include vaccinations, if given, for: Anthrax, Diphtheria-Tetanus, Hepatitis A, Hepatitis B, Herpes Zoster (Shingles), Human Papillomavirus (HPV), Japanese Encephalitis, Measles, Mumps, Rubella, Pneumococcal, Polio, Rabies, Rotavirus, Typhoid, Smallpox, Yellow Fever.

2. If the person has for any reason traveled in Africa, the Middle East, or the Far East and received vaccinations not listed above, note vaccination given, date given, location visited, and length of stay.

3. If person takes influenza vaccines, list date last given any reactions.
   a. Seasonal flu vaccination
   b. H1N1 (indicate drops or shot)

F. **Surgical History**
1. List most recent surgery first.

2. Give date of surgery, date of release, hospital, surgeon, kind of surgery, and outcome.

G. **Nonsurgical Hospital/Skilled Nursing Facility Stays**

1. List most recent stay first.

2. Give date of entry, date of release, facility, physician, and reason for stay.

H. **History of Illness**

1. Past Major Illnesses: Major childhood illnesses, cancer, other; when they occurred; course of illness and its treatment; after-effects being experienced now.

2. Current/Ongoing Illnesses/Disabilities (other than dementia which is listed in section IIIC): Give year began, course of the illness and its treatment (cancer, kidney disease, other), and outcome.

FINANCIAL AND LEGAL INFORMATION

Section I: Financial and Legal Advisors

A. **Advisor List**

1. Include the contact name and phone number for accountants, attorneys, financial planners, insurance agents, brokers, bankers, trust account managers, and any other professionals used for financial and legal purposes.

B. If two or more professionals are used for the same general purpose (e.g., Uncle Pete uses three accountants), indicate what each professional does (e.g., Uncle Pete uses Lou Harriman as an accountant for tax purposes, Bob Levin for business accounting for a small business Pete owns, and Sheila Dowd for handling Pete's trust).

Section II: Legal Documents

A. **Documents Prepared**
Indicate which of the following critical documents the person has, which professional prepared it, and where it is stored. If you or another

person is identified in the document as a designated trustee, surrogate, etc., list the name of the person designated as well.

1. Will
2. Living will
3. Trusts (revocable, irrevocable, living, etc.)
4. Healthcare surrogate
5. Durable Power of Attorney (business only)
6. Durable Power of Attorney with medical authorization

B. **Missing Documents**
If a document from the list has not been prepared, what plans are being made to prepare one? When will this be done and what professional will assist in the process?

Section III: Personal Papers

List the following personal papers, including identification/account numbers or description, issuing agency, and location where copies are stored.

A. Birth Certificate

B. Passport

C. Adoption papers

D. Naturalization papers

E. Official state picture identification

F. Marriage certificate(s)

G. Divorce decree(s)

H. Social Security card

I. Social Security benefit records

J. Medicaid card

K. VA and military records

L. Property deed(s) (list addresses)

M. Rental agreements, leases

N. Warranties and service contracts

O. Automobile titles (list make/model, year, vehicle identification number/ VIN, whether owned or leased (give date lease expires)

P. Insurance policies and cards for long-term care insurance, supplemental insurance, catastrophic and income replacement coverage, etc.

Section IV: Tax Records

Indicate the years and location of the following tax records. (Note: The records you should keep and the time you should retain them vary, typically on the period of time you may be subject to audit. Check with your accountant or taxing agency.)

A. Federal

B. State

C. City

D. Property tax/similar taxes

E. Other taxes by type

Section V: Pre-Need Funeral Plans

For each plan:

A. List the funeral home's name, address, and phone number; whether plan is prepaid or not, irrevocable or not, cash value amount, and name of person(s) plan is for. Has individual made all planning arrangements (chosen the casket and monument, set up perpetual care, where is each plot located, etc.)?

B. Indicate location of copies of the agreement(s) for the plan and cemetery deeds.

C. If there is no prepaid plan, describe plans for paying when need arises.

D. If no planning for funeral costs is in place, plan now.

Section VI: Credit Cards

A. List the name, account number, account ID or PIN or password for card use, current expiration date, location of card.

B. List name and website (URL) for issuing company, customer service phone.

C. If managed online or auto-pay has been set up, include user name, password, security questions and other security responses, minimum payment, if any is set, and which bank account or other payment option the auto-pay is charged to.

Section VII: Checking/Savings/Banking

A. **Checking Accounts and Debit Cards**

   1. List bank, branch used, type of account, account number, debit/ account PIN, location of checks for bank account, customer service number.

   2. If managed online, list website (URL), login information (user name, password, security questions, other security information).

B. **Savings Accounts**

   1. List bank, branch used, type of account, account number, debit/ account PIN, location of checks for bank account, customer service number.

   2. List name and website (URL) for issuing company, customer service phone.

   3. If managed online and/or auto deposit(s) into the account has been set up, include user name, password, security questions and other security responses, minimum payment, if any is set, and which bank account or other payment option the auto deposit is drawn from.

Section VIII: Bill Payment

A. **Automatic Payments**

   1. List the name of company, mailing address, customer service number, account number, or identifying information.

2. If managed online or auto-pay has been set up, include user name, password, security questions and other security responses, minimum payment, if any is set, and which bank account or other payment option the auto-pay is charged to.

B. **Paper Payments**

1. List the name of company, mailing address, customer service number, account number, or identifying information.

2. Include payment due date and forms of payment accepted.

3. Where are prior receipts kept?

4. Are any accounts past due or delinquent? If so, what steps can be taken and when to address the problem?

Section IX: Investments

A. **Certificates of Deposit**

1. List bank name, branch used, mailing address, certificate numbers, and locations of certificates.

2. If managed online, list website (URL), user name or other identifying information, password, security questions and other security responses.

B. **Brokerage Accounts**

1. List company name, address, phone number, account number, type, and broker's name.

2. If managed online, list website (URL), user name or other identifying information, password, security questions and other security responses.

C. **Stocks and Bonds Not Held in Brokerage Accounts**

1. List company name, address, phone number, account number (if one is provided for management purposes), type, and name of individual or office in company to contact with questions.

2. If managed online, list website (URL), user name or other identifying information, password, security questions and other security responses.

D. **Annuities**

    1. List company name, address, phone number, account number (if one is provided for management purposes), type, and name of individual or office in company to contact with questions.

    2. If managed online, list website (URL), user name or other identifying information, password, security questions and other security responses.

E. **IRA(s) and Other Retirement Funds**

    1. List company/bank name, address, phone number, account number (if one is provided for management purposes), type, and name of individual or office in company to contact with questions.

    2. If managed online, list website (URL), user name or other identifying information, password, security questions and other security responses.

F. **Pension Plans**

    1. List name of source (company, government entity, etc.) and contact information including name, address, phone number, account number (if one is provided for management purposes), type, and name of individual or office in company to contact with questions.

    2. If managed online, list website (URL), user name or other identifying information, password, security questions, and other security responses.

Section X: Property Records

A. List property address, date purchased, whether paid for or mortgaged, and location of deed.

B. If the property is mortgaged, list name of mortgage holder, type of mortgage, date will be fully paid, due date of payment, form of payment accepted, address for sending payment, and customer service phone number.

C. If managed online, list website (URL), user name or other identifying information, password, security questions and other security responses.

D. If there are special payments and terms, such as balloon payments, describe.

E. If the property is rented/leased to other parties and is managed by a management company, note the name and contact information for the company, fees for management, length of contract, and monthly income from the property.

Section XI: Insurance

A. **Health and Life Insurance Policies**

1. List type of insurance, the issuing company name, account or member identification number, group number (if any), access PIN, if required to access information by phone, current expiration date, and location of card.

2. List website (URL) for issuing company, customer service phone number.

3. If managed online or auto-pay has been set up, include online account number, if any, user name, password, security questions and other security responses, minimum payment, if any is set, and which bank account or other payment option the auto-pay is charged to.

B. **Other Insurance**

1. List type of insurance, the issuing company name, account or member identification number, group number (if any), access PIN, if required to access information by phone, current expiration date, and location of card.

2. List website (URL) for issuing company, customer service phone number.

3. If managed online or auto-pay has been set up, include online account number, if any, user name, password, security questions and other security responses, minimum payment, if any is set, and which bank account or other payment option the auto-pay is charged to.

Section XII: Inventory

A. An inventory can have many uses. It provides a list of personal belongings and the approximate value of what is owned in order to determine insurance coverage needed. It can provide documentation when claiming an insurance loss due to a theft, storm damage, or other covered loss. It can be used to plan replacement of property that is approaching its projected end of usefulness. And, of particular importance in planning for family caregiving, it can be useful in establishing net worth and in planning the distribution of an estate. If your loved one wants particular people to have specific personal items, as you conduct the inventory it can be helpful to label those items with people's names and make a note as to who should get them so that distributing them is easier when the time comes to do so.

B. If possible, the inventory should include the description of the item, an estimated value, its date of purchase and/or installation, and its location. For some items, such as household appliances or jewelry, it is advisable to retain purchase receipts or contracts and a record of payment. For other items, such as antiques, it might be appropriate to have a professional prepare an evaluation of condition and current value.

C. It is useful to have both a list on paper and photographs or a video recording showing all items.

D. It is advisable to have more than one copy of both paper lists and of photos or videos kept in different locations. For example, one copy of everything can be a hard copy kept by a family member and another copy can be stored on a computer in another location.

E. Total the value of all items and determine whether the inventoried items constitute a countable asset in planning.

F. Review the level of insurance on inventoried items (Too little? Too much?) and whether insurance coverage should be adjusted. A consideration: Full coverage may be too costly in relation to the person's income. What are the options for coverage?

Section XIII: Document and Property Storage Not Listed Above

A. **Safety Deposit Boxes**

For each box, list the bank (or other location), box number, method of access, location of the key, who is authorized to access the box. Give a general description of contents.

B. **Safes**

For each safe, list the location, provide the combination, or give the location of the combination.

C. **Computerized Records**

If the person maintains a set of backup disks for key documents, medical records, etc., give the location of the disks and date of last update. If records are stored on the Internet (cloud), list services used, passwords, and PINs.

D. **Storage Units**

List the address, unit number, and location of the key (or combination or location of combination, if a combination lock is used). Give a general description of each unit's contents.

Section XIV: Websites Regularly Used to Answer Important Questions

It is useful to keep a record of websites used frequently to answer important questions, for example, about healthcare issues, stocks, etc. List the website addresses and, if needed for access, the user name and password for each.

Section XV: Other Information

A. Is there other information about the person's life history, lifestyle, health, legal matters, etc., that could be useful? Be sure to provide it.

B. Does the person have an online personal health record? How is it accessed? Where are prior x-rays, scans, blood tests that may be in your loved one's possession?

MONTHLY INCOME AND EXPENSES

Carefully examining monthly income and expenses at the outset provides the best chance of containing expenses, stretching funds over the long-term, and preserving assets. List the items below that apply. Include most recent or monthly average dollar amounts (estimate where necessary).

Section I: Income

- Salary/wages (by each employer)
- Social Security
- Pension(s)
- Annuities
- Stock dividends
- IRAs
- Bonds
- Mutual funds
- Rental property income (by property)
- Partnerships
- Other income

Total this income

Section II: Expenses

- Rent/Mortgage payment
- Home/Household insurance
- Home maintenance
- Condo/Association monthly fees
- Property tax
- Telephone
- Electricity/Natural gas
- Water/Sewage/Trash
- Auto Loan/Lease payments
- Auto insurance
- Gasoline
- Food
- Healthcare and related insurance

- Employer provided group plan contribution
- Dental
- Medicare supplemental policies
- Long-term care policies
- Disability
- Other
- Healthcare expense not covered by insurance
- Prescriptions
- Medical supplies
- Treatment co-pays
- Dental/Vision/Hearing
- Over-the-counter medications
- Medical transportation
- Life insurance
- Child support
- Alimony
- Recreation and entertainment (hobbies, memberships, dining out, sports, movies, plays, other events)
- Charitable donations and gifts
- Direct caregiving expenses (e.g., cost of in-home paid caregiver not covered by insurance)
- Incidental caregiving expenses (e.g., gifts for facility staff at Christmas)
- Miscellaneous

Total these expenses

**Subtract Total Expenses
from Total Income
to determine Net Income.**

These lists are comprehensive but not exhaustive. Therefore, items that may pertain to you or your loved one may not be included. The items listed are memory joggers. Be creative in considering what else should or might be included.

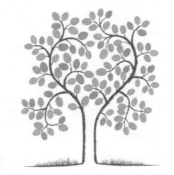

7.

Thinking About "What If . . . ?"

An important planning step in family caregiving is finding out what a spouse, loved one, relative, or friend wants and needs when care is required. Even if care is underway, it is not too late to discuss preferences and needs. As family caregiver, it's critical to find ways to create understandings about "what ifs" and balance them within the planning framework.

Overcoming Objections

You may have to deal with what Mom or your chronically ill daughter is willing to accept and where she draws the line. Sometimes all or a portion of needed care is rejected by the person requiring care. Someone else who is in denial (or who has other interests, such as saving money) objects to needed care being provided. It may also be necessary to take firm action if what the person needing care wants is at odds with the care and assistance needed. Sometimes the person needing care (or someone else in the family) demands that some form of dangerous or unneeded care be provided. When disagreements arise, you may wish to seek professional advice. Also, professionals in the field of disability, aging, and eldercare can provide highly specialized support.

If faith is important to a person needing care or family members, involve clergy and spiritual advisors to help everyone deal with stress and emotions. Keep in mind that most clergy and spiritual advisors have not been formally trained in family caregiver practical problem solving, and religious training does not automatically bring caregiver skills with it.

Anyone taking on caregiving must give careful thought to capabilities for contributing in terms of time, money, and required level of physical and emotional commitment. Think about life beyond family caregiving. Deciding on your family caregiver role requires self-sought and self-taught education. If you have not already done so, investigate the following to help determine your capabilities and capacity:

- Obtain personalized advice from all needed professionals.
- Learn about the current status of your loved one's care needs.
- Access definitive resources for care.
- Get good information to make better and wiser care facility choices.
- Search Internet sites to identify quality sources of information and qualified providers and then be prepared to test the reliability of sources and interview and scrutinize providers before you make any selection. Your loved one cannot do this, and you need to understand what is really needed. A pretty outside does not mean good care on the inside.

Think about life beyond family caregiving.

- Develop sufficient skills to effectively evaluate live-in help or unsupervised workers and be prepared to contract with them with specific information about what is expected.
- Become knowledgeable about background checks, references, and how to prepare and ask interview questions.
- Ask yourself whether you are the right person to interview potential paid helpers. Would another person be more effective at getting the right answers and judging whether a candidate is the right candidate? Should more than one person participate in interviews?
- Educate yourself on important durable medical equipment (DME), e.g., wheelchairs, Hoyer lifts, health aids, and other devices useful for maintaining your loved one's independence.

- Research home care resources to deal with potential issues when you need an agency. Not all are alike; some have their own employees, and others simply select individuals from a registry under a contract.
- Discover providers for formal assessments and third-party evaluations.
- Recognize the limits of your knowledge of legal, financial, and insurance issues and documentation and seek appropriate professional advice.
- Seek guidance in finding, accessing, and assessing community-based public and private resources.

Along the way, you and Dad will have to work together to find the answers that work best for both of you. Because family caregiving is dynamic and evolving over time, you both need to recognize that change is part of every family caregiving relationship, and both of you will need to adapt to those changes.

Change is part of every family caregiving relationship.

Understand that what worked yesterday may not work today. The old ways you handled care may need to be adjusted to meet changes in need and severity to ensure that the best options for care are being used to solve both old and new problems.

Also, you need to understand the essential distinctions between what is a normal part of a person's stage of life and age and what defines disability or disease. For example, you need to be able to distinguish between what is normal aging and what is illness—and help Dad and Mom to understand which is which.

It is not unusual for Dad to postpone or delay an annual medical checkup or seeing a specialist whether a problem is big or small. Why? Because Dad is afraid of what the doctor may find and say or does not fully understand alternatives and the implications of what is said. Elders like Dad may lack awareness or trust in changes and new techniques in medicine and the health sciences because of old stereotypes, myths, and prior assumptions. This lack of understanding or trust may leave him afraid to act.

You need to be prepared for the fact that Mom may resist taking the steps that seem to make the most sense to preserve her health and safety, independence, dignity, and quality of life. Mom may be reluctant to accept her aging and infirmities and perceive any illness or condition as a sure sign of old age and approaching decrepitude. It is important to make Mom understand that normal aging is not a disease; it is a process of life; a continuum that started the day she was born. That same perception can lead Mom to assume that, regardless of available treatment, a medical problem is inevitable and an unchanging result of aging, so why bother to treat it?

 TIP: An excellent book on the subject of conversations with older loved ones and relatives is *How to Say It to Seniors: Closing the Communication Gap with Our Elders* by David Solie, MS, PA.

When You Are Already Giving Care

When care is needed, you may encounter more objections to providing assistance than before the need arose. Regardless of age, it is only human for someone facing illness or disability to ask, "Why me?" Fighting loss of independence or the perception of isolation inevitably detracts from the joys of living.

Do not dismiss objections as unreasonable or representing a loss of decision-making ability. As a family caregiver, you must first ask, "Why? Why is Mom objecting to the help being suggested?" Think about the difficulty she may have in simply admitting that she needs help or is dependent on you for anything. Even a child, just learning what independence means, can fear its loss. Always imagine your reaction if you were the one needing care.

People of any age will react to change, especially sudden change and the undeniable realization that things may never be the same again. Some ignore it, hoping it will go away. Others get angry at themselves, fate, and God. Still others look for scapegoats—someone or something to blame. Some may insist nothing has changed at all, while others run away, literally or emotionally.

Do not dismiss objections as unreasonable or representing a loss of decision-making ability.

Whatever form resistance takes, remember the instinctive reaction of any human being is to fight to keep the status quo for better or worse.

Focusing on the decision-making process affecting care is essential. Planning at the outset, even for care in a major clinical setting (e.g., hospital, nursing home, rehab), can be easier if all aspects can be discussed. The issue goes beyond illness and setting to what may happen after that.

The need to manage expectations is critical. Without defeating a person's desire to get better, sometimes a small reality check is needed. For example, your eighty-six-year-old grandmother has been square dancing every Wednesday and Saturday since she was old enough to dance. One Saturday on the dance floor, she slips and breaks a hip. At the hospital, the surgeon says, "I am putting in a pin; you will be as good as new." When she leaves the hospital and goes into the rehabilitation center, the physical therapist says, "I will have your range of motion back to where it was in no time." Naturally, when everyone tells her that she will be "good as new," Grandma's expectations are that she will be dancing in a month or two.

However, when two months have gone by and she is still in pain, it still hurts to walk, and she has not been back on the dance floor, she feels she has been misled and feels miserable, angry, and resentful. She did not get the promised results: "You will be back like new in no time." Grandma is the victim of unmanaged expectations.

It would have been far simpler for you, a few days after surgery, to better manage her expectations by telling her, "Grandma, the doctors are pleased with your surgery and we will see how physical therapy goes, but keep in the back of your mind that things could take longer than everybody is telling you. Plan on waltzing a while before you square dance." This posture makes expectations more manageable without taking hope away from Grandma for a full clinical recovery.

Also, particularly where adults are concerned, but even sometimes when children are involved, someone who needs care may have major concerns about expense. A child may feel guilty about parents spending so much time and money. If Dad has limited income, limited resources, and/or limited insurance, he may resist care. The fear of assets being depleted is a legitimate concern. However, many times people believe that care is more costly than it is, and therefore do not understand the costs nor how those costs will be covered. It helps if everyone involved understands what things cost and how the bills will be paid. Preplanning can be helpful in relieving concerns because everyone has a better idea of how things will be handled.

Relying on home care from strangers may also create anxiety. The people who provide care will be strangers and may have different ethnic, cultural, or educational backgrounds; they could be older or younger or of a different gender. Remember that when someone enters your comfort zone you may feel vulnerable, and it is easy to see why Mom, who has a cognitive problem, or your young daughter, who only knows her parents, might be fearful or anxious or object.

Also, keep an eye open and ear out for *passive* resistance. Dad may not directly state his objections to some recommended action. He may say nothing when you tell him his house is dirty and needs a professional housecleaning or agree to bring in a cleaner, but then take no action.

Overt resistance comes in many forms, including the following:

- Lack of acceptance, "I don't need any help. I can do it myself!"
- Unrealistic acceptance, "I can get all the help I need from my family."
- False acceptance, "I would do it, but it's a waste of my hard-earned money!"

You need to learn to read between the lines, to recognize the unspoken story, so you can better understand where your loved ones are coming from. Regardless, you have to have respect for their decision. When a decision could result in a lack of care or obvious potential problems, you have to have a plan for how to overcome them. Young or old, no one wins a heated argument involving entrenched fears, values, or assumptions. There is no magic word that will resolve these kinds of disagreements. However, there are ideas and approaches that may work, and you have to think about things not previously considered.

Practical problem solving involves all kinds of fixes. Some work for only a few days, as if you are using safety pins, a little glue, and thumbtacks to hold the plan together until a more permanent, a more effective arrangement can be worked out.

What Can You Do?

- **Be patient.** Many decisions do not have to be made instantly. If a life is not in immediate danger, a few hours or days will not matter.

- **Try to understand the underlying causes.** Taking time to think about why Dad resists may help you realize that while Dad may be genuinely stubborn, there is more to his saying "NO!" to help than may be obvious.

- **Ask direct questions in response to objections.** If Uncle Ed says, "I don't need to pay somebody to do something I've done all my life," ask, "Uncle Ed, are you worried about the cost?" If he answers yes, you and Uncle Ed need to discuss ways his concerns can be alleviated. Also, while he may have always done something, the question has to be asked, "Is he physically able to continue doing it?"

- **LISTEN carefully.** Do not interrupt. Do not judge. Do not dismiss. Do not always assume that you are right and Dad is wrong simply because he is being stubborn. He may not have heard all the information you heard, may have processed it differently, or listened selectively only to what he wanted to hear.

- **Use supportive language.** "I can imagine how tough this must be for you. I am just trying to make it easier for us to work this out. Let's huddle like we always have and figure ways to make things better. We will both be a lot happier if we think this through together."

- **Show your belief in your loved one's good judgment.** Your brother, though ill, needs to feel he is capable of good judgment, but remind him that because his need for care affects everyone, other key people need to be involved in decision-making.

- **Look for compromises and mutual ground.** It takes time to build a trust relationship for problem solving. No one has to win; everyone just needs to have input, so no one loses.

- **If the discussion becomes strained, take a break.** State clearly that there is a problem to solve and you have to talk about it until it is resolved, but everyone can take a break for a day to consider each other's position.

- **Set a firm time to meet.** "We will talk again tomorrow night. Is seven or eight-o-clock better for you?"

- **Keep things in perspective.** Is winning an argument more important to you than understanding your wife's need for help? If your answer is yes, chances for success in convincing her to make a decision to do it *your* way are lower.

- **Remind everyone that the decision affects everyone,** not just the one who needs care. It affects you—your independence and quality of life—and everyone else in the family and their independence and quality of life.

- **Emphasize the importance of collaboration.** Tell Dad he's important, and by collaborating the family will find a way to resolve the situation, as you have always done in the past.

- **Consider that full-blown action may not be needed now.** There may be useful alternatives that can take you a little further along the way to the final goal. For example, as a result of an auto accident, your forty-one-year-old sister has trauma-induced frontal temporal lobe dementia (FTD) and has now come to live with you. She cannot stay by herself during the day while you work but is okay when someone is there to monitor her, and she can maintain a fairly normal home life. There is a local adult day care that has an innovative program for people with FTD that she can attend some days, and on some days your other sister will be able to stay with her.

Most of the time the people involved will agree to do homework, assemble paperwork, and gather information for the Plan. However, some adults may resist, dismissing your request as premature or as an invasion of privacy. You may feel compelled to respect this need to protect personal dignity and privacy, but remember that refusal may pose a real threat to the person's future independence. You must be prepared to overcome your reluctance to be tough in spite of your feelings of respect for your parents or any other person for whom you are acting as family caregiver.

Adults may fear becoming a burden, but in order to plan you need to know the details of legal, financial, and other matters. You are raising the issue now because people need to be prepared in the event of a temporary incapacity. Dealing with a parent (or any independent adult) can be frustrating, especially if this is your first encounter with your parent in your role as his or her family caregiver. Remember that in a parent's mind and memory, you are likely still a child who depends on him or her for care.

Similar issues based on fear of losing dignity and independence and being dependent on others arise within any reasoning person—even a child. Be sensitive to such fears. Explain what may be coming and why some steps must be taken now. If you do, you can greatly reduce fear and negativity for the person who needs care.

Do not over-manage your own expectations or assume you will always prevail. There are generational differences. Things important to you at fifteen or twenty or fifty-five haven't the same importance to Dad at eighty-two. Priorities and issues are very different based on generational milestones. For example, do not project on others how you feel about nursing homes; you're not the one going. It is more important to keep Dad's perspective and where he is in his life.

Finally, in many cases, a child can and does have a perspective on what he or she would like to do and can participate as an active decision-maker. Do not assume your child who is ill does not, or should not, have input on and an opinion about the kind of care he or she should have.

 TIP: These discussions need to be handled with patience. For example, if you are talking to your parents, make it clear that you are not there as your parents' child, nor as part of a parent/child relationship, but as a potential family caregiver. If Mom and Dad are competent, position your role based on your awareness of potential problems. Relate issues to them by telling what you know from friends and relatives who are dealing with similar problems. Make sure they understand that this is a group discussion dedicated to resolving potential problems. Avoid being overbearing or judgmental. But remember, being a family caregiver is a different role with different control and conflict issues.

You cannot please everyone all of the time. Regardless, some things must be done from the outset to prevent problems. The earlier potential disagreements are put on the table and you know each other's position, the easier it will be to reach an acceptable decision. Again, if Dad is a competent adult, he has the absolute right to decide what he wants to do or not have done.

TIP: Get Mom's and Dad's wishes in writing regarding the creation of essential legal and financial documents for end-of-life events and similar discussions. Do not wait because, while today they are mentally competent, their mental competence may become an issue tomorrow, and that will bring into question their ability to execute such documentation.

Getting Things in Order

Involving Other People and Technology

The Plan gives you a central place to assemble known information and to identify information you need in order to fill in missing, critical-decision elements. In particular, working out the Plan will enable you to identify where you need human help to make things work. Also, whether there are too few people to help or because technology may offer greater efficiency, consider how technology can do the work humans have traditionally done.

People Resources

To sustain successful family caregiving, you have to develop a support system. It takes time to identify the roles of the people and resources needed and to make sure everyone's responsibilities are clear, but doing so is part of an effective Plan.

Making decisions about who could be involved and whether to involve them is a complex issue. Participation can be loaded with potential pitfalls arising from prior relationships, finances, outside obligations, location, sibling indifference, multiple marriages, and more. Regardless, there may be many people who can and would help. Do not limit the list to just family. Dad's friends from the Moose Lodge may be just as willing to get him out of the house to visit his cousin, Marion.

- Anyone having regular contact is a potential helper. For instance, the regular postal carrier who delivers Dad's mail could report that his mailbox has gone unemptied and is crammed with letters.

- If someone has shown concern and offered to help, do not be afraid to ask them for help.

- Give a key and access to Dad's house to good friends.

- Even neighbors who do not want to get too deeply involved can be enlisted to report that something seems out of the ordinary. They may be willing to exchange phone numbers with you so that in emergencies they can contact you and you can contact them. Having this kind of support is especially important if you are a long-distance family caregiver.

- Third-party services can be hired to call several times a day to speak to and check on Mom.

- Family members can check by phone or visiting, whether they are siblings, nieces, grandchildren, cousins, etc.

- Check with Dad's clergy to see if they can provide assistance, if what is requested is clearly defined and not too imposing. Some religious organizations have volunteer groups than can provide companionship, run errands, and assist in other ways.

- Contact local service organizations to see if they have volunteers who can call or visit.

- Contact local community centers (youth centers, senior centers, family centers), community service organizations, and hospitals to get suggestions for care resources.

- Local merchants can be valuable resources. Identify individuals who have regular interaction with Mom (e.g., the beautician or local shopkeeper accustomed to seeing her on a regular basis). Often, they are first to notice unusual behavior or absence. They also may want to help Mom in any way they can. Take time to locate them and share your concerns.

- Identify businesses, including restaurants, that deliver services "on demand." You can arrange with local merchants to prepay by credit card (including a tip, if appropriate) for services like plumbing and painting to get work done in Uncle Paul's house and for the preparation and delivery of meals he likes to eat. If you make arrangements to prepay for a service or meal and have something delivered, be sure to tell Uncle Paul you have made the arrangements, everything is prepaid, and the tip has already been paid so he will not pay again. Always call to make sure the service or meal was delivered as planned.

Identifying potential human resources and allowing them to help is an important job. It never hurts to ask. It might surprise you who says, "Yes," and the level of support they are willing to provide.

For long-distance caregivers, finding unrelated but caring helpers living near Mom can be helpful. It may require a few weekend visits to identify who those helpers might be.

Be resourceful, but remain vigilant. Letting people into Dad's home without having much background knowledge of them can pose a risk.

And remember, no one, including you, has to do everything. The idea is to identify the right people to help when small but crucial tasks arise. For example, if Mom has a cat, is someone willing to feed it on short notice if she goes into the hospital?

Using Technology

In the past, human beings were the only available "tool" for monitoring a person's well-being or a patient's conditioning, diagnosing an illness, and reporting on changes that needed to be addressed. Today, and even more so in the future, technology offers options for doing some of those tasks in ways that may save time and money, but more importantly that free human hands to perform other tasks.

There are technological tools that can be attached to telephone and Internet systems that allow constant monitoring of physiological changes; battery-operated devices that detect and store information as a person wears them during normal activities from which data can be uploaded for analysis; and many other applications that exist or are in development. These tools allow continuous local- and long-distance monitoring, and even long-distance diagnosis. Many devices are in use or being developed in the healthcare field that have a potential for changing the way healthcare is accessed, monitored, and delivered.

The idea is to identify the right people to help when small but crucial tasks arise.

Technology also can allow us to maintain personal contact. Installing a computer with Internet services, a camera, and a microphone; providing cell phones; and using other equipment can make keeping in contact easier and provide greater peace of mind when you are not actually there. Technology can allow your loved one to reach you quickly and easily. However, keep three issues in mind if you want to use technology: 1) just because you can use a computer does not mean that Aunt Ethel will be able or willing to do so; 2) using technology needs to be a joint decision, and its use cannot be perceived as "spying" by your loved one; 3) keeping devices running may pose technology hurdles, and costs may exceed available funds (e.g., accessing reliable satellite service in some areas and expensive costs for data transfer).

Calling a Family Meeting

When Grandma needs care, every family member is affected, but not everyone may want to be part of the response. Some people may distance themselves from the situation and disappear at times of need. Others come forward and are eager to help. Others will help but need to be encouraged to do so. One key to successful caregiving is for everyone to be involved in planning, and, of course, in providing care at some level. Many hands make light work. Gather everyone's ideas about how best to meet care needs.

Experts, especially eldercare mediators, suggest calling a family meeting as early as possible. A family meeting provides a forum for everyone to be aware of needs and how best to meet those needs. It is also useful to seek professional advice about legal, financial, and clinical issues to help everyone gain better insight and to seek additional advice as needed over time.

The family meeting's focus must be, "Everyone is here because we are concerned and want to help." Some family members will be involved hands-on; others may provide financial and other indirect support. In the end, everyone needs to understand that care needs will change over time, and those giving direct hands-on care will need reasonable relief.

Everyone needs to understand the meeting is not about them, but about Mom's need for care. Mom's independence, dignity, and quality of life are paramount. Without considering these three elements, no mutually effective Plan can be built. That does not mean that Mom will automatically get everything she has said she wants. It does mean her well-being is of the highest concern. For example, if institutional care is required, overruling Mom's objections will not be easy to face, but what has to be done, has to be done. Regardless of roadblocks you can anticipate in the future, keep in mind that the goal of the family meeting is to assess family support.

Who Attends?

Do not exclude anyone from the meeting; even a young child can help. Also it may be appropriate to include close friends. However, people may be more forthcoming with offers if Grandpa is not present. After the meeting, you can discuss with him what happened.

Let Grandpa know that everyone is working toward the best possible Plan to provide him with the care he needs in the setting he would want. Try to include Grandpa in subsequent planning and decision-making. Again, assuming Grandpa is competent, he has the final say if his health and safety are not jeopardized. One issue you need to confront may be Grandpa's former decision-making role. He may resist change (change can represent loss of independence or create anxiety in anyone), and you may have to work with him to help him understand why the change is necessary. Even people in the early stages of something like Alzheimer's may still be capable of contributing to the Plan and, if not significantly impaired cognitively, should still have that chance. You may have to work harder to find alternatives to form a Plan that works for Grandpa, but if he accepts the Plan he will cooperate rather than resist. However, be prepared—the family may have to make decisions for his own good that might make him unhappy. Making hard decisions is one price paid in being family caregivers.

Children needing care have the same right to be informed. If their situations are properly explained to them, they can contribute. They may make major contributions by explaining how they feel, what they believe they need, and what makes them most comfortable. For a child, not knowing can be more frightening than knowing; remember that expectation management is important for everyone involved.

Also, do not forget to include a brother and sister who may become *de facto* caregivers when adults are not around. Their insight and perspective may be very helpful. Just as there are differences in the viewpoints and perceptions contributed by a fifty- and a seventy-year-old, a nine-year-old may have a perspective more in line with what his twelve-year-old brother may need, think, or expect than their thirty-five-year-old parents. Everyone affected should be asked to share.

Finally . . .

Keep the lines of communication open. Avoid family meeting "melt down." Anything beats hearing a final "No!" Let everyone know you will continue your research and will bring back findings for further consideration. State firmly that if the situation has to be resolved, then it must be resolved to everyone's reasonable satisfaction. A stubborn "No!" from any one person may lead to unacceptable outcomes.

Grandma needs to feel a sense of involvement and control over her life and destiny, especially when her independence is threatened. As mentioned, perceptions of what is important vary at different stages of aging, and, whatever your good intentions about fulfilling the needs and wants of Grandma may be, her perceptions of what is needed may be different.

Keep the lines of communication open.

Spousal caregiving is very different from care offered by adult children to their parents, not in terms of what or how it is being done, but with regard to the relationship. Each partner is accustomed to the other playing a specific role in the relationship. If the partner needing care is no longer able to play that role or wants to play the role, but is either incompetent or unrealistic, the other partner may have difficulty taking on the role of decision maker.

TIP: Adult children are very aware of the acute care medical system because they use it, too. When an older parent says, "Ask the doctor what to do," which is normal for an older adult to say, there is a tendency to do just that. However, nonclinical family caregiving is typically outside a doctor's area of expertise and comfort zone. Once outside their areas of expertise, doctors are no longer the experts. It is rare to find a doctor in practice who has ever considered nonclinical family caregiving issues in planning care for patients. Many doctors dealing with family caregiving challenges in their own families are no better at it than you. Doctors ask doctor friends for advice, too, but like you, when it comes to family caregiving, they "don't know what they don't know."

People have confidence in their regular doctors. Doctors are competent authorities for clinical issues. If your doctor cannot answer a nonclinical question on which a clinical issue decision or action depends, he or she needs to understand that you are exploring more options. When you have assembled the options and alternatives, perhaps then the doctor can contribute opinions.

More Tips for Creating a Positive Family Meeting

- **Do not expect things to go smoothly.** Emotions are likely to run high as past issues are raised in response to this call for help. You do not need people backing away because of hurt feelings or family conflicts with others.

- **Sometimes it is helpful to have an objective third party conduct the meeting.** A third party may be better able to handle emotional responses, provide support, and keep the focus on the Plan. A certified family mediator, family counselor, social worker, or trusted family advisor—someone with professional expertise—might best serve as facilitator.

- When talking to individual family members, **focus on what their immediate contributions can be**. Some people have money but no time, or time but no money. Others may have a history with Dad that makes it difficult for them to offer hands-on assistance.

- Do not forget to **consider social customs that can affect what people are willing to do, versus what they are able to do.** For example, if you and your family live in Iowa, what your sister will do for your Mom and what your brother will do may differ because of social or cultural biases, rather than the physical ability to perform a particular task. Your brother may live with Mom full time, but if Mom has to be bathed or have help going to the toilet, he may come up against internal constraints that make him unwilling to help her perform those tasks and her to accept his help. Your Dad may absolutely refuse to have your sister or any other woman bathe him. Let ideas for solutions come from group members.

- **Leave doors open for change.** As primary caregiver, accept what is offered now with no judgment about whether or not it is enough or fair to everyone else. Later, the reluctant person may be more forthcoming with support. If not, the time to discuss why a person is unwilling or unable to do their fair share is not at the family meeting.

- **Talk about available resources.**
  - How can available funds best cover care for as long as possible?
  - How will resources be supplemented?
  - What are possible options?
  - What financial responsibility do family members now bear for costs of care? What can they afford to bear?
  - Do not overlook normal expenses (e.g., travel, telephone, time taken from work) for people who help.

- **Having the beginnings of the Plan makes great sense.**
  - Do not just assemble a stack of incomplete information clustered into a series of "maybe this or maybe that" options.
  - Prepare a workable outline to comment on and discuss; if you do, it is more likely that productive conclusions can be reached.
  - A draft or outline of the Plan can contribute immensely to a sense of order.
  - Even a draft Plan can project "what ifs," like staying home or not staying home, sources of funding, and who is the primary caregiver for certain events.

- **Include physically unavailable family members in the family meeting.** Talk to them in advance; get their ideas and comments; report on their contributions at the meeting. See if they can attend by conference call, web cam, or live chat.

- **Remind everyone that there are all sorts of ways to help**, including, for example, the following:
  - Out of town? Come visit or invite Grandma to visit, giving the primary caregiver a break.
  - Young children can be responsible for small household chores, such as walking a pet, emptying trash, bringing in the mail, so their mother can concentrate on caring for their disabled brother.
  - Others living nearby can do chores, such as yard work, outside maintenance, and driving a grandparent to and from the doctor.
  - If someone has trouble offering help with direct care, perhaps they could be responsible for routine tasks—grocery shopping, paying bills, making medical appointments, or dealing with paid help.

Before the meeting closes:

- Repeat or summarize what everyone has agreed to do, writing down the summary as you go. Note areas of needed care that have not been covered. Ask again for suggestions for providing those services. Have someone make copies so participants have copies *before* they leave.
- Everyone needs to make a commitment to hold family meetings on a regular basis, perhaps every six to eight weeks at first. Set a date for the next meeting *before* adjourning.
- As soon as possible after the meeting and using your notes as a guide, start to prepare a typed Plan. Identify gaps and summarize people's commitments then send the document to family members who need to know the Plan. Putting the Plan into a formal format gives it more impact and importance.
- As you prepare the Plan, you need to consider the ability of others to read and use the Plan once it is on paper. Does everyone read and speak a common language, English, for example? If not, how are those who don't speak English going to use the Plan? Does everyone who speaks English know how to read? Can they read easily or do they struggle? Do you need to take time to review the plan with someone verbally or through a translator? Do you need to help another person develop visual or aural cues to remind him or her of what has to be done and when?

Starting the Discussion About Caregiving Needs

The earlier you discuss family caregiving needs, the better. When issues under discussion concern possibilities that still seem years away, people tend to be more open about their real feelings. Even if your wife is only thirty years old or Grandma is well advanced in years, do not be reluctant to broach the possible need for care. You may be surprised to find people who may need care someday are not only willing to discuss these matters but are relieved you raised the subject. However, there are some important considerations when you start to discuss caregiving, whether you expect it to happen tomorrow or years from today.

- **If you sense reluctance, discuss your own plans.** Talk about the Advanced Directives you have signed (or plan to sign). Suggest that appointing someone as a Durable Power of Attorney made good sense for you. Talk about your thoughts on care when your time comes. Ask your wife for her thoughts, opinions, and ideas.

- **Timing is everything.** If sixty-seven-year-old Uncle Ed is going through a particularly tough time, use the opportunity to open the discussion. Discuss stories in the press or on TV about Parkinson's disease and family caregiving (they are everywhere). Don't plan to accomplish everything in one discussion. No crisis? Then, take your time and wait for the right mood and moment to discuss concerns.

- Before any discussion on the need for care begins, stop! Consider Mom's feelings. If she has always been basically healthy and independent, now having to rely on anyone for anything will be upsetting for her. If Dad managed people in business, he may resist you managing his life. If Grandpa always handled finances, Grandma may be concerned about assuming those responsibilities. Your older brother may have problems entrusting serious life matters to you because you're the kid who couldn't keep your room clean or tie shoelaces without his help. Your niece may think because she is still young and able that planning ahead is not important.

- Hopefully, your relationship with Mom and Dad has matured into one of equality, and they respect you as an adult and a decision-maker. However, when the chips are down, anticipate that Mom or Dad will revert to their old (established) parenting personalities. Other relatives may respond negatively to protect themselves against threats to their independence and autonomy.

And, to ensure better outcomes, try the following ideas:

- Acknowledge to Dad that being faced with the need for care is something neither of you would have ever wanted.

- Acknowledge how tough it is to even consider the idea of needing help when Mom has always been active and helpful to others.

- Remind your son who was injured in Afghanistan and needs assistance that his willingness to consider help now could substantially postpone the possible need for more intensive help later.

- Show that your wish is to be supportive and open, rather than to be the person in charge.

- Choose a time when emotions are likely to be under control, a time when you are both rested and are not likely to be interrupted.

- If there is difficult information to be shared or decisions to be made, let other "higher authorities" deliver that news (physician, clergy, lawyer) while you offer support, options, and solutions.

- Solicit input. Ask, "What do you think, Uncle John?"

- Ask questions not easily answered with a simple yes or no.

- Enlist advice about a particular service provider from Mom's trusted friends or neighbors; they may know someone who used the provider and for whom the service made a positive difference.

- Are there major changes to be made? Take things one small step at a time. Ask your sister, who is becoming more impaired by MS, to try the service or idea for a set period of time. Let her know she's doing it for you, for your peace-of-mind and out of respect for concern for her well-being.

The need for your help and assistance can begin gradually or happen suddenly. The better you are prepared, the better you know your options. Making knowledgeable and timely decisions creates peace-of-mind for you and for everyone else involved.

 TIP: Using others' experiences as examples is always helpful. If talking about assisted living, ask, "Dad, why do you think the Murphys, who have lived here as long as you, decided to move to an assisted living facility?" Listen carefully for clues. If Dad says, "They couldn't manage the house," ask him, "What would you consider doing if you were in the same circumstance?" Don't force answers; just plant seeds and see if they grow into Dad's ideas.

 TIP: If you know someone must relocate to a smaller place that is handicap-accessible, an assisted living where he or she will have ready care, or another institution, never try to make the other location sound better than home or where the person lives now.

For example, when Aunt Clara has lived in the same home for decades and is surrounded by years of memories in a place where significant events in her life occurred, nothing else is going to sound better. Your best answer may be, "Clara, you are staying in the house, but we have to fix it up." Then, tell her you will get estimates for the work to be done, for necessary equipment, redoing the bathrooms, adding wheelchair ramps, installing the new furnace, replacing the roof, etc. Once Clara finds out what making the place both livable and safe can be, she may decide, "That's too much money to spend on this old place." Or if she wants it all fixed, remind her that she has to have money to live on and pay for other things that might come up, so ask how she wishes to pay for the repairs.

In the end, after careful thought and consideration, the only explanation for the change that will ring true is that under the circumstances the new environment will provide what that person needs to be safe and well cared for. It may take time to reach that understanding, but in the end it is the more important consideration.

Knowing When Care Is Needed

How do you know when help is needed? What are the signs in children or adults who cannot clearly speak for themselves or do not realize that something is wrong?

Are you prepared for the hospital call in the middle of the night, or something less dramatic? Anyone can suffer a traumatic event or a sudden disability. A simple accident or seemingly minor illness can result in a long-term recovery period. Chronic illnesses and disabilities can develop in a more subtle fashion; there may never be a call in the middle of the night to alert you.

Consider your Uncle Max who for years has run an isolated fish camp in Minnesota. He appears fine from a distance and says he is fine on the phone. He is

Learn early warning signs that signal a loved one's need for assistance.

"Mr. Independence." You invite Uncle Max to visit his sister (your mother) and send him a ticket. When he gets off the plane, you can see that he seems frail, does not walk with confidence, and seems a bit confused.

It is obvious that Uncle Max is experiencing a wide range of signs and symptoms that may signal a need for intervention.

Whether you are concerned only with yourself or have people around you that you care for, adults or children, you need to learn early warning signs that signal a loved one's need for assistance. Some of those early warning signs are the following:

- Difficulty walking, managing stairs, finding words, completing thoughts, remembering details, directions, or names.
- General complaints of feeling tired, sick, or chronic pain.
- Changes in physical appearance: weight loss or gain, changes in skin tone, bruising, or neglect of personal hygiene.
- Changes in mental outlook: loss of interest in normal activities, lack of energy, mood swings, or depression.
- Difficulty in managing routine tasks: socializing or playing well with others, doing homework, bill paying, meal preparation, household chores, or work-related activity.

Take Steps Now

Even when care or assistance seems years away, take steps now to make the transition easier.

- **Be aware of any chronic conditions or hereditary illnesses** that could precipitate a crisis and the need for care (e.g., diabetes, heart disease, cancer, dementia).
- **Prepare a master file** of all medical records and family history. (See Chapter Six for suggested content.) As a parent of a dependent child you can easily work with physicians and other providers to develop your son's record.

If needed for Dad, he will have to request the documentation, or you will need to have a signed Durable Powers of Attorney with Medical Authority or a Designation as Healthcare Surrogate in order to receive records from attending physicians, nursing facilities, or hospitals. Advanced Directives should expressly address your loved one's issues. Such documents can always be changed, but it is critical to have them in place *before* the problems start.

- **Know your Grandma's physicians, financial and legal advisors, and others to be called** when help is needed. If needs are imminent, let all concerned parties know whom to contact and how they can be reached.

- **Get professional assistance** for any additional information to help you prepare for when care is needed.

- **Be familiar with community service options** where Grandpa lives (especially if he doesn't live in your community), including such local services as home healthcare agencies, adult day care centers, other care facilities (assisted living, rehabilitative, and nursing care), and local support groups.

- **There are numerous government agencies** for children, adults, and the elderly (e.g., the local Area Agency on Aging)—for almost any special population—that can send information about specialized care, meal delivery, transportation, in-home chore assistance, translation services, and so on. Also ask about local family caregiver support groups.

Be Aware and Be Wary!

If your husband has been diagnosed with a potentially disabling chronic illness (e.g., Lou Gehrig's disease [ALS], diabetes, arthritis) using the best resources can certainly help. To be an effective family caregiver, you need to be familiar with the symptoms and conditions of the illness or disease involved and aware of what to reasonably expect. Some information will not apply; some may be right on target. When you better understand options, it is easier to make wiser decisions. Be careful in choosing sources of information. Rely on nationally recognized organizations, such as the Arthritis Foundation or the National Institutes for Health. Well-recognized websites provide valuable information about managing diseases, new findings, research programs, and drug trials.

Notwithstanding what you learn, every clinical healthcare decision should be discussed with your husband's doctors. Do not try anything not previously prescribed or recommended by anyone not completely familiar with your husband's full circumstances.

Keep your support circle and family up-to-date. Sharing recent information provides a regular basis for soliciting needed assistance. A time will come when you need to take a break and get some respite.

The reality of care is that sometimes your loved one does not respond to conventional therapy or respond the way you would want. Do not let your concern lead to you making poor decisions. Families get desperate and will try anything. If you see claims of a cure or a superficial article about something that "holds possibilities" in the newspaper, a "cure" promoted in a flyer, sketchy or exaggerated information on the Internet or TV, or hear something passed along word of mouth, **be skeptical!**

Brief articles about possible cures come out all the time with misrepresented content, or that discuss possibilities that will take 100 years to make a reality, if they ever become a reality. If a "cure" was that good and that true, you would hear about it from responsible scientific and medical professionals, not presented in an advertisement. Any disease or condition that becomes a hot topic, as is the case for cognitive issues and dementia such as Alzheimer's disease right now, also

> **Do not let your concern lead to you making poor decisions.**

becomes an especially popular topic for this kind of advertising and reporting because very little help is available and desperation knocks out objectivity.

Be a cautious consumer, especially at times of stress or frustration with conventional treatment. Call a Center of Excellence in the condition (for example, the MD Anderson Cancer Center at the University of Texas or the James Buchanan Brady Urological Institute at Johns Hopkins Hospital for prostate issues) and ask what the medical professionals know about the "miracle cure."

You Are Planning, So What Else?

- When you are caring for **a special needs child**, the Plan should include directions for what happens if you are not around to provide care. Seek the assistance of a qualified disability attorney to prepare appropriate documents. Seek other professionals to consider financial resources, insurance, and other essentials. A trustworthy and responsible adult must be chosen to serve as a guardian should you not be around.

- If your loved one is **an older but active adult**, preparing needed legal documents and beginning to plan now are steps that will save everyone a great deal of frustration later.

- If Dad receives **Social Security**, the amount received should be verified. The local Social Security office should be contacted to request direct deposit of checks into the appropriate bank account.

- Also, check the **website www.Medicare.gov for Medicare coverage**. If inquiring by phone or mail for Dad about Medicare, the staff will ask Dad to verify that you are authorized to inquire on his behalf to access information. In emergencies, and when Dad is not unavailable, Medicare will normally offer a "courtesy period" to help assist in the problem. Long term, you need supportive documentation. Get it prepared, signed, and sent.

- **Everyone of legal age needs a Durable Powers of Attorney** for financial and healthcare decisions in the event of incapacity. Everyone's situation is different, and requirements vary from state to state. Using a generic example as a substitute for a formal document prepared by a qualified attorney is risky. For example, documents prepared by an elder law attorney will address Mom's particular needs. This is especially important in accessing public benefits (Medicaid, VA) as the document needs much greater specificity than the typical Durable Powers of Attorney.

  Note: The Durable Powers of Attorney for Healthcare and for Advanced Directives are usually separate documents. They also may vary from state to state in terms of necessary language or citations to specific statutes or laws.

- The wisdom and good sense in having a **qualified legal professional prepare documents** is that the documents will follow state laws and will clearly set forth in legal terms individual wishes for how to deal with serious illness and for end-of-life choices.

- **When family resources are limited** to a single Social Security check, a single wage, a few dollars in savings, or limited life insurance, even a short-term illness or an accident can be financially devastating. Even when resources are apparently nonexistent, it is vital that a family examine options in the family and those available in the community. Planning ahead can make it possible for even severe illness or a long-term issue to be easier to bear.

- Even with the best Plan, when care for a **catastrophic illness or care over a period of years** is needed, a lifetime of savings can be spent quickly. Discuss purchasing catastrophic care and long-term care insurance to help cover costs of care at home, in an assisted living facility (ALF) or a skilled nursing facility (SNF). If it is too late to add to personal resources, or if required care is unaffordable, public benefits may be the only potential option for support.

- **Review assets**—property, stocks, bank accounts, and other holdings—to mutually determine the best circumstance to protect your spouse (and children) if you are physically or mentally incapacitated. Joint ownership of accounts may ease access but may complicate qualifying for other benefits, so get professional advice.

- **A use analysis of all future spending** may be required. A use analysis is provided by professional planners who assess present and long-term needs. Such analysis is quite different from services provided by estate and trusts attorneys, who prepare documents usable upon death, or from traditional financial planners, who prepare documents to preserve assets for heirs upon death. These economic planning professionals work to assess present and long-term needs while you are living, plot the rate of using assets, and make sure anticipated care needs can be properly funded. They will help you understand whether other funding sources, such as public benefits, may be required. This planning is critical in an age of increasing longevity.

- If you anticipate a **need to access assistance** (Medicaid, Railroad, Social Security, or VA benefits), *before* you move or retitle assets, discuss this with an elder law attorney. Care has to be taken to avoid violating "gifting" laws or making assets "countable" when redistributing them. You need a professional's advice so you do not defeat the Plan's financing strategies.

- If you anticipate needing Medicaid for Mom, remember that **Medicaid is a loan** from the government. Assets need to be protected from being subject to recovery on her passing. Consult an elder law attorney to make sure assets conform to the Medicaid rules and regulations in Mom's state.

- If a Dad is **reluctant to tackle** important issues, demonstrate their importance by telling him you are doing the same things for your own financial and legal protection.

Every relationship you have with another person is a dynamic relationship. Elements in your lives change daily, sometimes obviously, sometimes subtly. The same is true for family caregiving; every family caregiving experience is as unique as a fingerprint, is subject to rapid change, and will uniquely affect your Plan.

Never assume yesterday's situation is today's, or that today's will be the same as tomorrow's. Even with the best Plan, plans can go astray. Managing these events is like running a military campaign. There is an overall objective and individual plans are put in place to reach that objective. A good family caregiver, like a good general, knows that he or she cannot win every battle but firmly believes the war can be won.

 TIP: Having the Plan lets you think about "what if" events, essential to implementing flexible, workable, long-term care strategies. Remember the comparison that planning for caregiving is like planning a road trip? Imagine you want to take a road trip from Miami, Florida, to Seattle, Washington. Would you just jump in the car and drive North and West and hope to get to Seattle? Or would you check the route, search online for maps and directions, and lay out the whole trip? Would you check your car and make sure it's in good shape; plan rest stops, places to eat and visit; and schedule time to relax from the drive? That's making a plan.

The point of the Plan is to give you some idea of where you are going in family caregiving. You cannot stop medical problems from occurring, but as a family caregiver, you can prepare for the social, psychological, practical, and emotional problems that may arise. Just knowing those roadblocks may be out there takes the element of surprise out of what is a very blind trail.

Planning for Financial Needs

In planning ahead for family caregiving, you will consider assistance offered by state and local governments. However, local services may be limited, take time to put into place, or be unfunded or unavailable.

Providing care can be expensive for Grandma and for you and those supporting the care effort. You need to be aware of ways to guide care and assist in determining how best to manage expenses effectively.

Medical Expenses

Clinical care is a commodity, just like a car. Do not be afraid to shop around. Every clinical services user needs to be a knowledgeable consumer. Being knowledgeable is part of what makes you an effective advocate. Ask questions. Know the reasons for care recommendations. Ask about costs. Challenge options. The more you know, the greater the likelihood the care you arrange will be both cost effective and medically effective. Doctors are constantly negotiating rates with Medicare, Medicaid, major medical insurers, and private payers. Do not be afraid to negotiate rates and services with the professionals, including medical doctors.

Ask questions. Know the reasons for care recommendations. Ask about costs. Challenge options.

While it is not easy to challenge time spent on services, do not be afraid to say that fees are beyond Uncle Ed's ability to pay. Can accommodations be made? This is the same bartering technique used every day in business; do not be afraid to try it in the medical setting.

Always read the bill for services rendered, especially after a hospital or rehab facility stay. Even if a service is covered by Medicare, Medicaid, major medical insurers, and private payers, that does not mean you should not check it carefully. Overcharges and nonexistent services drive up everyone's costs.

Treatment

Regardless of age or circumstance surrounding the need for care, healthcare providers deliver services at payment rates acceptable to insurers. Every insurer has its own rates, and you must make sure physicians, specialists, and facilities that will be used are part of your insurer's network and have agreed to provide services for those rates if that insurer is to cover the costs.

For example, you need to be sure that Mom's doctor accepts Medicare assignment—that is, accepts payment according to the rates Medicare pays. Further, if Mom is being sent for a series of tests or procedures, try to negotiate for a discount since the provider knows that payment will be made for several tests. The cost may be "cheaper by the dozen." Also, be sure her supplemental (gap) insurance or Medicare Advantage Program covers the procedure(s) she needs. Each policy differs in terms, referrals to specialists, length of stay, or limited use of facilities. Each insurer may differ in what they include versus standard Fee-for-Service (FFS) Medicare.

Prescriptions

All prescriptions should be discussed with the prescribing physician. Ask for suggestions on ways to cut expenses. Let the doctor know cost is a concern and ask whether he can prescribe less expensive or generic alternatives.

Generics are chemical equivalents of branded drugs. However, be aware: Manufacturing varies by location (worldwide) and the binders, fillers, and coatings used in generic drugs may differ from those used in the branded drug. While less expensive, these variants may have side effects that negatively affect certain users, making the branded drug the only choice.

Shop at pharmacies that offer generic drugs at flat rates, which are typically less than $10 per prescription. Try getting ninety-day supplies by mail to cut costs. Take advantage of local discount programs that may be negotiated by county or city governments or for special groups of users (e.g., healthcare cooperatives, membership organizations).

Finally, know the rules for drug coverage and copayments under your insurance plans. Insurers more or less have three lists of drugs: the brand names they cover, the generics they cover, and the drugs that do not fall in either list and are not covered. The insurer may require ninety-day prescriptions, monthly authorizations, and so on. Know the rules before purchasing a prescription. Do not be surprised by a pharmacist telling you the drug prescribed for you or your loved one is not covered.

Remember: People covered by Medicare are required to have Medicare Part D, the prescription drug program.

Tests and Diagnostic Procedures

When a test or diagnostic procedure is ordered, ask about the necessity for the test and what it costs. While every test has value when used correctly, many may not be necessary or needed as often as recommended. There is no harm in asking.

If you know that the same test has been done recently by another doctor, hospital, or healthcare professional, tell the doctor and ask whether that test's results are recent enough to satisfy the requirements of a proposed new test. Using those results could save time and money, and asking does not mean you are questioning medical need or the doctor's judgment.

Testing for Cognitive Impairment

Testing to determine whether there is a cognitive issue is a necessary step. Cognitive issues are of increasing concern worldwide. Research is leading not only to an increased understanding of the nature of cognitive disorders but also to the differences between one type of cognitive failure and another, as well as one type of dementia and another. For that reason, we are including this section in the *Manual*, the only section on a specific disorder.

Never assume confusion and memory loss mean a person has dementia, including Alzheimer's. Confusion and memory loss can be caused by medications, inappropriate dosages (accidental or prescribed), hormonal imbalances, alcohol, a wide range of clinical issues, and the infamous "senior moment."

First bring the behaviors to the attention of your loved one's physician, who should then conduct a thorough medical examination to ensure that physical or drug issues are not causing the symptoms you see. If they are causing the problems, steps can be taken to reduce or eliminate the effects.

There are a number of tests that can be administered to determine a person's basic cognitive capacity. Such tests, which are called psychometric tests, may be administered by a physician, social worker, psychologist, or other healthcare professional who has been trained to administer the test and interpret the results. Evaluation of test results is subjective and highly reflective of the scorer's training, interpretation, and inherent biases. It is recommended that several tests be used, including two of the quickest tests which are also the most commonly given at this time, the **Mini Mental State Examination (MMSE)** and the **Clock Test.** If there is any doubt about the results, do not be afraid to go to another provider for retesting. The ultimate authority is typically a neurologist or neuropsychologist who specializes in these matters. Your general practitioner may not be the most appropriate person for the final determination.

The Mini Mental is a brief test that offers a quick and simple way to quantify cognitive function and screen for cognitive loss. It tests the individual's orientation, attention, calculation, recall, language, and motor skills. This is often the first test given *but should not be the only test given.* The test focuses on answering a number of questions, such as the following:

1. **Is the patient "in the moment" (knows the time, dates, his or her location, etc.)?** The test taker is asked basic questions such as "What day is it?" and "When were you born?"

2. **Does the test taker have "recall"?** The tester speaks three words to the test taker (such as apple, penny, table), who is asked to recall the three words that were spoken and repeat them back to the tester. At the end of the test, the tester asks the test taker to repeat the same three words (that is, recall them). Another example is that the tester may ask the test taker to count backward from 100 by 7s (i.e., 100, 93, 86, 79, 72, etc.).

3. **Is the patient oriented visually and spatially?** The tester presents the test taker with a picture of, for example, two overlapping boxes and asks the test taker to draw the same picture.

4. **Poor performance (i.e., a low score) on the Mini Mental may indicate cognitive problems are present,** but it will be necessary to administer additional, more involved psychometric and brain scan tests to determine the extent and nature of those problems.

Next Step Tests

If the outcome of the Mini Mental indicates there may be a problem, the next step is referral to a neurologist, who will determine whether there are physical changes that could account for the poor score. For example, has reduced blood flow (as in vascular dementia) caused brain damage?

Most neurologists also have a mental health specialist—a neuropsychologist, a psychiatrist—administer a body of psychometric tests that have been proven to test cognitive ability or deficit, such as that shown in Alzheimer's. For example, a poor score on the Clock Test, again one of a number of tests that should be given, is considered a good indicator that a person has Alzheimer's. The tester asks the patient to draw a clock face (i.e., draw a circle and place the numbers one through twelve in the standard position of a clock face) and then to draw the large and small hands to indicate a specific time (e.g., twenty minutes past three). A person with cognitive issues typically draws the clock face inaccurately and, therefore, scores poorly. The circle may be flat like a pie pan seen from the side or drawn as a ragged oval, the hands may be outside the circle, there may be only one hand—there are many variations. People who score poorly on the test likely have deficits in the part of memory associated with words, knowledge, and understanding.

The results of the neurological exam and the psychometric testing also may show an older person is experiencing a normal aging process. The results may also present a clear picture of cognitive problems a person of any age may be experiencing and help define the type of problem (Alzheimer's disease, frontal temporal lobe dementia, concussion-related dementia, vascular dementia, and so on). Knowing what the results indicate also enables us to anticipate future issues.

Research and Drug Tests

Physicians who serve as Principal Investigators in government-approved research studies, such as the testing of a new drug approved for human testing by the FDA, have to meet stringent standards to engage in testing. Their research is closely monitored and can lead to significant breakthroughs that benefit many people experiencing a chronic or debilitating illness or disability.

If your loved one is offered the opportunity to participate in such a study, it is worth considering. First you should verify the credentials of the physicians conducting the research. If things check out, your loved one may benefit from the treatment being investigated. However, you need to be realistic and manage expectations. A drug that showed good results in a test using animals may not work in humans. There may be side effects. And, keep in mind that in some studies only some of the people participating actually receive the treatment being tested, while others receive a harmless but useless substitute (a placebo). Regardless, you may consider the potential for benefit worth the risk. Remember: Human testing requires humans—without doing human testing, we will never make meaningful progress in treating any form of presently irreversible dementia.

Surgery

If surgery is suggested, ask whether there are less invasive alternatives, such as drug or physical therapy. Surgery may be a wise choice but not the only choice. There may be an acceptable, non-surgical option/intervention, but if you do not ask, you (yes, you; remember that you may also be your own caregiver!) could unnecessarily undergo a risky, expensive, and invasive procedure. Check the National Institutes of Health website at **www.nih.gov** or major disease/illness organization websites for the latest alternative therapy(ies). Consider all the options carefully; at the same time, understand that options and alternatives may not be viable in your particular circumstances.

Never be afraid to ask for a second opinion. Most insurers will pay for second surgical opinions. It is just as important to them to know whether the procedure is essential or about the availability of less costly alternatives. If a physician presents surgery as the only recourse, but you are getting conflicting opinions from other qualified sources, consider switching doctors. Contact your insurer to discuss it with a trained advisor. Remember, surgeons do surgery; that is their expertise and source of income. It is important to get second or even third opinions from non-surgical specialists in the condition, rather than accept surgery as the only recourse. For example, a cardiologist is not a heart surgeon and may provide non-surgical expertise to better understand what is involved and help you make a wiser decision.

> **Caution: Obvious life and death decisions should not be put off simply to seek another opinion—delay may be very dangerous.**

If surgery is indicated, contact the insurer in advance to see if all costs will be covered and, if not, what extra expenses you can expect. Many insurers, including Medicare Advantage Programs, require prior written permission before surgery is done and may also restrict use of out-of-network physicians and surgeons, hospitals, and outpatient clinics.

Be aware that you may not see your doctor while you are in the hospital after the surgery is done. Many insurers and hospitals use a "hospitalist" to oversee hospitalized patient's clinical care. These hospitalists are qualified physicians and are paid to render good medical advice and move the discharge process along. However, they work for the insurers and hospitals, not for you! That means sometimes things are overlooked. For example, the hospitalist may say your elderly next door neighbor, who looks to you for advice but not healthcare, is ready to go home after heart surgery. You know she has no one at home to help. You can and should ask what plans are being put into place to provide critical home care support that should be paid for by the insurer. When you (or someone you care for) are in the hospital, it is very important that you find out who are your patient advocate and your discharge planner. Both of these people know what the bigger picture is for being discharged. Avoid surprises—contact them early.

LEGAL CONSIDERATIONS
A Few Words of Caution Regarding Legal Forms

If you need legal documents such as Durable Powers of Attorney, contracts for service, or wills, be very careful in using forms from the Internet or the local office supply store. The details of state-specific law vary widely and cannot be easily addressed by a generic form or by what some publishers claim are state-specific forms. Moreover, your need is not a generic need; it is very specific. Even online legal sites, which theoretically could update material daily, may not offer the state-specific information needed to address the circumstance you need to consider. The Internet is a source of useful information that you can use to gain knowledge and weigh options, but do not depend upon it as the final determiner of how you should handle a particular legal situation.

Seeking Advice

Specialized law for children, elders, and other special populations should never be left to a generalist. There are attorneys who specialize exclusively in issues affecting special-needs children, the disabled, older people, veterans, and family caregivers. Always look for board certifications in a specialty practice.

The protection of children's rights is complex, laws vary drastically by state, and addressing any legal matter associated with children requires specialization. A specialist can address issues of guardianship, institutional care for children, special education programs, special trusts, and so on.

For older people, you need a legal specialist in Medicare, Medicaid, state-provided services, and veterans benefits to prepare for long-term care needs. These specialists, typically certified as Elder Law attorneys, can review and advise on enrollment in institutions, such as assisted living facilities, coverage, and fine print exceptions for long-term care and short- and long-term disability insurance. Elder law attorneys are qualified to address and also include in their practice specialized issues surrounding disabled veterans, children, and other special-needs populations.

Other resources for getting financial and legal advice may be local law schools offering legal aid service advice on critical issues. The local Bar Association may recommend lawyers with the necessary expertise or offer legal aid clinics on elder law and other issues. Local government offices, such as the local Area Agency on Aging, might be able to recommend advisors or provide helpful literature. (Note: Legal aid agencies typically deal with criminal matters and civil cases, rarely with other issues, but it will not hurt to ask!)

Areas That Should Be Addressed

Everyone should plan on how to address estate and other issues that require legal advisement. Estate planning is determining how and where you want to allocate your assets upon your death. Your Plan for your own care should recognize the need for that but should focus on what you will need for the next decades of your life past age sixty-five. The following basic issues should be addressed when working with a legal advisor:

- **Estate planning**, including establishing wills and trusts to protect estate assets.

- **Planning for incapacity**, including establishing parental rights, issues of guardianship, living wills, healthcare directives, and powers of attorney for health decisions.

- **Planning for benefit eligibility**, including Social Security Disability Income, Medicare, Medicaid, veterans benefits.

- **Contract evaluation**, when arranging care services from facilities, providers, or any other form of care. This is especially important when applying for acceptance into an independent living (IL) or assisted living facility (ALF). Contracts for ILs and ALFs are extensive and you may need the help of others to conduct a careful review and to understand what the facility does and does not offer. Do not assume you know! Laws governing both types of facilities differ from state to state, as does the level of licensure required by each state. Do your homework so there are no surprises.

- **Protection of property**, including review of all assets and property and how access (legal and physical) is permitted to designated representatives should Mom become incapacitated.

- **Pre-planned funeral arrangements**, including terms of payment and future care of the gravesite.

   Note: If you also plan to apply for Medicaid or certain veteran's benefits at some point, the document establishing the terms of the pre-planned funeral should be **irrevocable,** so it cannot be counted as a cash value asset. Ask the funeral director for a letter stating that the pre-need agreement is irrevocable.

Careful planning for financial and legal matters saves time, dollars, and frustration.

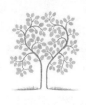

TIP: The *Manual*, including the list of documents and information that should be gathered (see Chapter Five), can help you organize and plan realistically for family caregiving eventualities. The more time spent planning before a crisis, the more manageable your family caregiving job will be.

TIP: Financial and legal planning is not inexpensive and must be budgeted for carefully. However, typically, the time and money saved by using these professionals will pay be repaid many times over. It is perfectly acceptable to discuss and negotiate fees.

UNDERSTANDING THE SERVICE NETWORK

There was a time when disabled or chronically ill people were either cared for at home (for elders, this is called aging-in-place), in a skilled nursing facility (SNF), **Regardless of age or need, people MUST largely rely on in-home care.** or in another institutional setting. Due to an ever-increasing shortage of SNF beds, today's system of delivering care for any population is challenging, complex, complicated, and confusing—in part because of society's assumptions, stereotypes, and myths regarding what it does or does not do.

Persons of any age may require significant medical support. Most elders prefer to receive care in the community and live at home. It is both a blessing and a curse that today, regardless of age or need, people MUST largely rely on in-home care anyway.

For elders in particular, aging-in-place is the care model for the twenty-first century. Currently, 37 million people sixty-five and up suffering chronic and long-term illness are cared for at home. And 60 percent of all long-term SNF beds are funded by Medicaid (and largely occupied by elders) with notoriously low reimbursements. No one is building new SNFs and many are now forty to fifty years old or older. There is little economic incentive to build new beds when reimbursement is at or below break-even levels.

Just like America's failing infrastructure of roads and bridges, chronic care facilities are also failing.

The acute care system (clinical care systems and hospitals) is trying to be the service delivery mechanism for long-term care, but much of the care needed is non-clinical. America is destined to have substantial delays and disconnects between what is needed and what can be delivered. The acute healthcare system has placed an unbelievable burden on the unpaid family care system. We all need to recognize that the work required of family caregivers may include clinical tasks we have never been trained to do.

Services and Programs

Notwithstanding limited institutional care, there are a variety of services and community programs available for care at home or in a community-based care setting. Names for services and community programs may vary from place to place, but functions will be similar. As aging-in-place predominates, additional categories of providers will emerge to help guide family caregivers and care for loved ones.

SERVICES

Note: Services vary from community to community. The services described below may or may not be found in your community, and services not listed may be available.

- **Chore Service** provides major household maintenance, such as replacing storm windows, screens, cleaning gutters.
- **Homemakers** perform routine tasks, such as cleaning, laundry, perhaps some personal care.
- **Home Health Aides** (HHAs) help primarily with personal care and activities of daily living (ADLs), such as bathing, dressing, toileting.
- **Certified Nursing Aides** (CNAs) have more training than HHAs, typically providing clinical chores in hospitals, SNFs, and home-based care.
- **Geriatric Care Managers** (GCMs) conduct care-planning assessments; identify problems; understand assistance eligibility and elder services; screens, arranges, and monitors in-home help services; review medical issues and offer referrals to geriatric and other specialists to avoid future problems and conserve assets; and also provide clinical crisis intervention to family and patients.

- **Registered Nurses** (RNs) are professionally trained and licensed. They monitor and manage care in hospitals, SNFs, and rehabs that requires high-level clinical assistance. RN numbers have dropped in the last few years. According to the American Nursing Association, in America between 2015 and 2020 estimates project a shortage of almost 1 million nurses, which will place enormous strain on healthcare delivery and make family caregiving even more complex.

- **Licensed Practical Nurses** (LPNs) are professionally trained and licensed. They provide front-line clinical home and facility care and oversee medications. There are fewer LPNs than RNs because the pay differential is significant.

- **Physical Therapists** (PTs) are professionally trained and licensed to help persons regain motor skills, adjust to changes in mobility, strengthen muscles, etc. Typically, rehabilitation is offered in SNFs following an accident, illness, or surgery. Physical therapy can be delivered in outpatient settings or at a patient's bedside. Under Medicare, you must be a hospital in-patient for seventy-two hours before being eligible for physical therapy.

- **Physical Therapist Assistants** (PTAs) are professionals trained and licensed to work in association with PTs and are the ones who actually do the physical treatment assessed and requested by PTs.

- **Occupational Therapists** (OTs) are professionals trained and licensed to help patients relearn basic ADL skills: dressing, cooking, bathing, toileting, and ambulation (moving) essential for persons who have had a stroke or crippling injury. This retraining plays a major role in improving quality-of-life. Under Medicare, you must be a hospital in-patient for seventy-two hours (which includes two overnight stays) before being eligible for physical therapy reimbursed by Medicare.

- **Speech Therapists** (STs) are professionals trained and licensed to work with speech and swallowing issues to retrain muscles and regain needed reflexes. Often speech therapists are essential for evaluating the patient's capability to swallow properly. Improper swallowing can lead to inhaling food and fluid into the lungs and getting aspiration pneumonia and/or severe choking episodes. Under Medicare, you must be a hospital in-patient for seventy-two hours before being eligible for speech therapy.

- **Social Workers** (SWs), **Licensed Clinical Social Workers** (LCSWs), and **Masters in Social Work** (MSWs) are professionals trained and licensed to help with care planning for future needs, filing insurance claims, determining eligibility for community programs, etc.

COMMUNITY PROGRAMS

Note: Programs vary from community to community. The programs described below may or may not be found in your community, and programs not listed may be available.

- **Adult Day Care** (ADC) is a community day program with trained staff for physically and cognitively challenged persons. They are typically limited to seniors and offer socialization, hot meals, and possibly professional services, such as PT. There is a shortage of quality ADCs, which reflects the rising prevalence of Alzheimer's dementia and chronic diseases. Some communities also offer specialized care for children who are at medical or emotional risk.

- **Respite Care** is a facility-based service offered for short-term stays (less than a month) to give family caregivers a break. Contact local SNFs, ALFs, or inpatient hospice facilities to see if they offer respite care. Smaller facilities (Board and Care) may also have respite availability. Note: Respite is typically a private pay service, but some long-term care insurers cover it.

- **Friendly Visitor/Phone Check Programs** are community volunteer programs. The volunteers check on the home-bound and offer companionship. This service offers a break from the daily routine for the family caregiver and people requiring care. Some communities have "Friendly Call" services; volunteers make daily or weekly calls to check in on the well-being of elders and the homebound and offer social contact.

- **Meal Programs** provide either home-delivered meals (commonly called "Meals-on-Wheels") or provide meals at centralized communal dining sites. Meal programs can be public or private services. The meal costs may be paid by users or funded by public funds. Public funding may be provided by the state and/or the federal government. State departments of elder affairs typically administer funds for elder's meals (sixty-year-olds and up) through local Area Agencies on Aging. Some local meal programs (typically privately funded or offered by local charities) are open to families and individuals under age sixty.

PUTTING CARE INTO PLACE

Before anyone enters your home to aid or assist with care, check the person's credentials. Do a background search or use only licensed agencies that complete employee background checks and reports and make sure that employees carry liability insurance.

It is very easy to create impressive sounding credentials, but the proof is in documentation that can be verified. Be careful! Many people with "shallow" healthcare backgrounds call themselves experts (in child care, geriatric care, and other special areas). Get references and call them. Ask direct questions about experience, nature of services, and charges. Verify the credentials of any service provider you use. Bringing

> **Before anyone enters your home to aid or assist with care, check the person's credentials.**

someone into your home to watch and care for an adult requires that you perform the same due diligence you would perform if you were trying to find a nanny for an infant.

If you are a long-distance family caregiver requiring supportive in-home care after hospitalization, GCMs and discharge planners are great resources. Contact them to help organize in-place home care services after discharge. (If you are not onsite, are not a primary caregiver, or are just helping out during someone's hospital stay, do not assume that hospital discharge planners are aware that the person lives alone and has no one to provide care in the home. Make sure that the discharge planner knows in-home care has to be arranged *before* discharge can be done.)

A word of warning: Most clinical facilities will not discuss patient care with anyone not legally designated as a healthcare surrogate or who does not hold Powers

> **Proper paperwork is essential, and copies must be in the patient's chart.**

of Attorney, without a release from the patient stating that the person is to be informed about his or her care. So, proper paperwork is essential, and copies must be in the patient's chart.

If the situation is grave, make sure **Advanced Directives and Living Wills** are also on file, making enforcement of Mom's end-of-life wishes easier to accomplish, without fighting medical bureaucracy.

If there is **no hospitalization or other need for care,** a private GCM can be retained for a one-time consultation on how to better deal with Aunt Edith. Locate qualified GCMs through the hospital discharge planner or contact the National Association of Professional Geriatric Care Managers (NAPGCM).

If post-hospitalization care is needed, be very prudent about choices and options. The ongoing well-being of Dad depends not only on where care takes place but also on who provides it. If long-term care insurance (LTCI) is being used, contact the insurer's case management department for a list of local, insurer-approved home care providers. At the same time, remember to verify coverage, reimbursement rates, co-pays, elimination periods, and caps on spending.

No matter who's involved, ultimately, you, if you are the designated family caregiver, are in charge of managing ongoing care. Note the word "designated." At some point, Grandma (and the family) elects a designated caregiver—the "go-to" person to handle emergencies and solve problems. The designated family caregiver receives the emergency calls, and when Mom insists, "... I don't need help and I don't want strangers in my house," he or she makes sure that care is provided.

Take the right steps when care is needed!

- **Step 1: Review the Plan.** Decide what is needed and who manages it so you can control other care.

- **Step 2: Encourage Mom or Dad or your disabled son to do as much self-care as possible.** Self-care maintains a person's sense of independence and dignity, as well as controlling and enhancing his or her physical ability to do things.

- **Step 3: Involve all relevant decision-makers to the extent each can contribute.** As the designated family caregiver, getting buy-in in advance can make your responsibilities less overwhelming and stressful.

CRISES

Your responsibility as an active family caregiver may begin when an emergency or unexpected change occurs. Successful emergency family caregiving depends on being prepared.

Regardless of your loved one's current health status, plan now for a possible emergency. This is especially important if the person you are caring for is elderly or has a history of health problems, such as when your son has a disability that leaves him vulnerable to infection.

In addition to having your caregiving Plan in place, you should also do the following:

- **Prepare an emergency information summary** (as recommended earlier). Print clearly—poorly written emergency information can be misread delaying assistance—or prepare the form on your computer. Print EMERGENCY INFORMATION in bright red ink at the top.

- **Prominently display the form** or put the form in an emergency pouch (sometimes provided by emergency services or available through medical equipment suppliers) on the family refrigerator. If you are not home or do not live with your loved one and a crisis occurs, EMTs and other emergency personnel are trained to look there for such a notice.

- **Place a copy** in Dad's car, Mom's wallet, a special needs child's book bag, and carry it with you in your own wallet.

- **Program emergency numbers for key people** into home and cell phones (yours, your child's, your parents'), so making a call for help is a button touch away.

- **Store critical information on a flash drive,** which is very portable (carried on a key chain or in credit card size in a wallet), and can be plugged into an onboard emergency vehicle or emergency room computer. A flash drive is an efficient way to provide medical history, care details, and copies of critical documents. (Be sure you take steps to protect sensitive information like Social Security Numbers; use passwords, blank out information, etc.) If a doctor keeps electronic health records (EHR), you may be able to download that information (such as x-rays, cardiograms, and prescriptions) for use by others and upload copies of things (such as legal documents and insurance information) into the doctor's files.

- **Update the Caregiving Plan frequently.** Always update information to reflect changes in prescriptions, medical conditions, insurance, providers, and other critical information. Old or inaccurate records make information useless, or worse, dangerous.

WHAT YOU NEED TO KNOW IN AN EMERGENCY

When an emergency occurs, whether you are waiting for EMT transport or are already in the ER, medical personnel are more concerned with giving care than answering questions. Be patient but vigilant.

We are accustomed to an admission being a matter of course in an emergency that appears to be something like a heart problem or when there is any question about health status. However, there are some hospitals now that have introduced something they call a "fast track," which is in reality a way of delaying admissions to determine what is going on with patients and, if possible, releasing them back to home without ever formally admitting them to the hospital.

Always determine whether the person has been admitted or is still under observation. You can even go to a bed on the floor for continuing observation without being admitted. For people covered by Medicare, that means the seventy-two-hour admission period under Medicare for post-acute benefits will not be triggered. Supposedly, this avoids inappropriate admissions, but it can mean that someone goes home who needs care but will not get it at home. Elderly people and the disabled are especially vulnerable due to potential inability to properly communicate or care for themselves. If there is any question about a person's condition, capacity to provide self-care, or having someone to care for him or her, make it clear that he or she cannot be released in those circumstances.

If Uncle Ed is admitted, ask for his personal property: wallet, jewelry, etc. Let the medical staff know about legal paperwork related to healthcare surrogacy if it is not already on file, or provide a copy immediately.

As the designated family caregiver, the alpha caregiver, make key people aware of your role in decision-making. Medical personnel will respond better if they know you are the main point of contact and can let other people know what is going on so they will not be repeating information to different people. You can keep the family informed and relay concerns and questions to medical personnel.

If you think you are not getting needed information, enlist help from social services or the patient advocate. If you are denied critical information, go to the highest levels and ask for the Administrator. Record all information and who gave it to you.

When you get to the hospital and your loved one is admitted, ask who the hospitalist is. Be prepared for things to progress rapidly, but you must keep cool. Be aware that the hospitalist may not be readily available because of large caseloads and works for the hospital and insurer and not you.

Once Mom is admitted, get answers to the following questions (also see "Questions to Ask the Doctor" in Chapter Eight).

If surgery is recommended, ask: Are there choices other than surgery? What are the expected surgical risks? What are possible results? What will the recovery time be?

If Mom is being treated and sent home, ask: What are home care needs? Who will provide that care? (Remember: The hospital staff may assume you are providing care when you are not.) What is the expected recovery or rehabilitation time? Will there be permanent after effects?

If Mom is discharged to a SNF or rehab, if you are able to do so, check it out personally. If you want a change made, get to the discharge planner who controls the placement. You need to make your needs known.

If Mom is hospitalized for an extended period, you need to take responsibility for routine details: getting mail, handling phone calls, stopping the newspaper, emptying the refrigerator, watering plants, feeding pets, etc. Others can handle these tasks. Use the Plan and develop a task schedule for others so you are free to handle more important issues.

Use the time to plan arrangements for home care. Work with the discharge planner, case manager, and physician to develop and understand their clinical plan-of-care. If formal services are required, immediately start to identify appropriate care agencies and personnel (they may already be in the Plan). Keep family members aware that their contributions to support and care are valued and important.

> *The information in the* Manual *is not meant to substitute for professional clinical information and care; rather, the* Manual *contains resources to help keep you focused in a time of stress. Consult the Plan. It is your map, but be aware of detours!*

The more you are seen as a source of quality information and as a good advocate, the better able you will be to maintain control, gain respect, and become welcomed by the medical professionals around you as a respected and functional part of the broader "care team." A cool head will gain more information.

TIP: Facilities are busy; everyone has a job to do. They have good and bad days, just as you do. Understand the roles of the people you are dealing with and their responsibilities they have for caring for Mom. Make sure you are dealing with the right person for the situation. Asking for assistance gains more help than demanding it. Facilities have corporate plans and protocols, must adhere to federal, state, and local rules and regulations, and also have to deal with personnel and facility operations. The world cannot stop because you want it to.

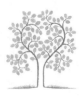

TIP: Being a successful advocate is part of the Plan. Pick battles carefully. Do not become known as the "person no one can satisfy." Having management and staff on your side makes difficult situations run much smoother. Be realistic. Hospitals, rehabs, and nursing facilities are not five-star hotels. Manage your expectations and your family's, but do not settle for something that is obviously inadequate or inappropriate, including staff attitudes.

8.

Practical Problem Solving

Your first task as a family caregiver is to gain a clear understanding of what you are facing so you can ensure medical and health needs are properly met. Effectiveness depends on your ability to anticipate needs and be prepared. Do not act before an emerging need has to be met, but do not ignore possibilities. Deal with first things first; that is why you have the Plan. The following sections are designed to help you summarize current needs and anticipate future ones.

Addressing Medical and Health Needs

A sudden event may not create the need for care, but preplanning is important even in anticipation that any ordinary day can bring change. You may find yourself in the role of family caregiver after a visit to Mom. You notice she is repeating the same story, again and again. You notice that Dad, who took great pride in his appearance, is not shaving or dressing much of the time. A visit to your sister reveals piles of unpaid bills and signs of household neglect, although she has always been meticulous about paying bills and household care.

Ask yourself, what prompted this need for assistance and care? Was it physical, mental, or emotional illness, catastrophic stroke or broken hip? Is there ongoing trauma because of the birth of a special needs child? Serious depression? Have a child's grades suddenly dropped? These are examples of changes you need to be vigilant about. Do not feel intimidated if you did not see the changes earlier. People are good at masking and covering up. It is easy for Grandma to say "I am fine" on the phone and sound like she always has even when nothing could be further from the truth.

But do not delay action when you do see the need. If the issue is medical, meet with or call Mom's primary physician and ask questions (see "Questions to Ask the Doctor" in this chapter). If Dad is admitted to the hospital, get an estimated length of stay, and find out who is preparing the discharge plan of care (DPOC) for his release. If the DPOC specifies home healthcare, get a copy of the plan in order to trigger long-term care insurance benefits (if any), as well as Medicare, Medicaid, VA, SSDI, and other applicable benefits, entitlements, or insurances. Ask for a review of medication: What changes were made in type, dose, and frequency, versus what he was taking when he entered the hospital? What prescriptions is he being given to take home? Should he continue to take the over-the-counter medications he was taking before admission with the changed or new medications?

Do not delay action when you do see the need.

Note: Regardless of the age of the person needing care, the major concerns of most caregivers will be how their loved ones will react to care provided by "outsiders," how the family caregiver will schedule care in relation to other commitments, how to pay for what is needed, and similar questions related to how to continue proper care irrespective of where care is provided or by whom.

In all non-routine clinical situations, have a meeting with all persons in charge. Introduce yourself as the designated family caregiver concerned about Uncle Ed's ability to maintain independence, dignity, and quality of life. Discuss your Uncle's physical and mental status and any changes you have noticed in behavior or outlook. Make certain you know how to contact them and how they reach you in an emergency or if a major change in clinical status were to occur.

Dad may be reluctant to provide emergency contact information to his doctor for fear of losing his independence or because he has an "I don't want to be a bother" attitude. Even though Dad has always been that way, what may have once seemed like a bother is now a necessity! You may need to take the initiative and insist on his listing you as an emergency contact.

When you are preparing the Plan, get the name of Cousin Tom's pharmacist and add it to the Plan. When Tom's medications are changed, the pharmacist may be more aware of potential polypharmacy dangers (taking multiple medications, both prescribed and over-the-counter, that may interact negatively with other medications or result in overmedication). The pharmacist should have a complete record of medications taken and provide information about side effects and risks. Some medications come via mail-order from the VA or another source, not the local pharmacy. Check all prescription bottles to identify both the medications and the sources. Pharmacists observe very strict privacy and HIPAA rules; so if you need information, give each pharmacist a copy of the Designated Healthcare Surrogate in which Cousin Tom named you as surrogate.

Grandpa's pharmacist has information that is important when trying to decide which Medicare Advantage Program or Plan D Drug Plan Grandpa should enroll in. The pharmacist knows Grandpa's prescription requirements and can help find the plan with a formulary (list of drugs covered) to meet his needs, reducing drug costs and avoiding non-formulary medication. However, the pharmacist cannot recommend a Medicare Advantage Plan D program because that is now considered steering, which is illegal.

Also, Grandpa may be taking numerous medications (prescribed, OTC, or herbal), but he may not share this information with all his doctors. Even when information is shared with them individually, doctors rarely speak to, or collaborate with, one another. Show each doctor the medications list. Ask if the medications each prescribed are still necessary and, if so, whether dosage or frequency can be lowered to help prevent drug interactions or reduce side effects and whether a generic drug can be used instead of a brand-name drug.

Reminder: Update the Plan when medication changes are made so the information can be found when you are not available.

When someone you are caring for appears to have a cognitive problem (e.g., confusion, memory loss), the cause may be a physical problem, medical issue, or adverse prescription reaction. Grandma should have a complete medical examination by a qualified professional. Ask whether depression could be at the root of her symptoms. Is she taking a medication you did not know about? Does she need a medication she is not taking?

 TIP: The government website www.MedlinePlus.gov reviews every medication, supplement, and OTC remedy legally sold in the United States. It is indexed, constantly updated, and explains product usage, dosage, and side effects. It also provides the contact numbers for poison control.

 TIP: Know which prescriptions your sister, who has MS, is taking. Check her prescription bottles regularly to see whether she is taking them as prescribed, too frequently, not frequently enough, or not at all. Check refill amounts and renewal dates. Do not wait until the supply runs out before you call the doctor for a prescription renewal; your sister may be required to have an office visit before the doctor will renew the prescription. You do not want to hear "No refill"!

Questions to Ask the Doctor

Communication may be a two-way street, but sometimes physicians and other healthcare professionals make assumptions about what patients and caregivers understand or need to know. You have a right to ask questions and ask them until you understand what is going on.

Always make a list of questions before you meet with the doctor. As the doctor talks, do not hesitate to interrupt with a polite "pardon me" to ask additional questions that come to mind. If you do not understand what he or she is telling you, it is useless information, and it is not rude to ask him or her to repeat something more slowly or in nonmedical terms.

If the meeting is too short to ask all your questions, let the doctor know you have other questions on your list that you need answers for. Set a time for a follow up phone call or get his or her email address so you can send the questions for response. Get a commitment for a prompt reply.

Here are questions you may need to ask:

- What is the diagnosis?
- What does that mean in layman's terms?
- What is the treatment?
- What is the prognosis (future outcome)?
- What else is my loved one facing?
- If there are multiple health issues, what are they?
- Is this a physical or mental illness? Both?
- Is more than one physician involved? Why? Get their names, specialties, and contact information.
- If so, are all physicians consulting and exchanging information?
- What new medications are being prescribed? Why? For how long? In what dosages and frequencies?
- What medications are being discontinued? Why?
- What are the side effects of the prescribed medications?
- Are you aware that my loved one is regularly using OTC medications? Alcohol?
- Are you aware that my loved one exceeds prescribed dosages/has multiple prescriptions for controlled substances (e.g., morphine)? Uses recreational drugs (e.g., marijuana)?
- Are there any concerns about continuing OTC medications while taking the prescribed ones?
- Are there lifestyle changes needed (e.g., a special diet, a special kind of exercise routine, more rest)?
- Are there symptoms to watch for indicating a progression or change in the diagnosed condition?

Overall Housing and Care Needs

Most people prefer care at home. Home is usually where we feel most secure, comfortable, and the least stressed. At the same time, home may not be the best place for care due to clinical, physical, and safety issues.

For example, you are still friends with your ex-husband Will who was recently injured in a car accident. You have taken on the task of caregiving for him, at least for the present. He is now confined to a wheelchair and will be for many months to come, if not permanently. He cannot get up the stairs, and all bedrooms and full baths in his house are upstairs (there is small half bath downstairs). Also, the neighborhood he lives in is not especially safe, and you have some concerns about his being vulnerable on the street and about your safety when entering and leaving his home. Still, he wants to stay in his home.

Home may not be the best place for care due to clinical, physical, and safety issues.

No matter how strongly you believe that your ex-husband, or any other person, should make lifestyle changes when faced with new care needs, you must be sensitive to the fact that home is home, and Will wants to stay. If he is competent, he is entitled to make his own decisions, even if those decisions are bad ones. Given this, how can you help?

- Survey the home's layout and condition. See the "Security/Safety/Condition Survey" in this chapter.
- Be realistic; can minor changes make major differences?
- Can a downstairs den convert easily to a bedroom with a simple bathroom?
- Can Will's wheelchair fit through the downstairs bathroom door?
- Is the stairwell wide enough to add a lift chair?
- If upkeep is a physical burden, can maintenance services be arranged?
- Explore taking in a college student or roommate for companionship and to share household chores.
- If location makes assistance hard to obtain, investigate formal live-in options for managing care.

Housing Options for Adults

Ultimately, staying in the home may not be possible. While hard to accept, the reality that facility care is needed following a catastrophic illness or injury eventually sinks in. Allow a little time for emotional adjustment before tackling the loaded topic of moving. Obviously, if care needs require immediate action, get the Plan and implement the care options.

For example, if Mom cannot return to her home, look beyond a stand-alone SNF or ALF and consider a long-term care/lifestyle community offering a more residential facility, one that is smaller and more inviting, with a homelike atmosphere. There are larger adult-only (ages fifty-five and up) continuing care retirement communities (CCRCs), which include independent living; assisted living; dementia care; and skilled nursing all on-site. Some are created for frail elders or those with dementia allowing them to live as independently as possible, but they are in an environment of supervision, peers, recreation, and social activities designed to preserve not only their quality of life but also their dignity and independence.

The best choice may be to have Mom live with you, the primary family caregiver. Before making a commitment, take time to fully consider the impact on everyone involved, especially when you still have young children at home. Consider how having your brother, who is disabled and in a wheelchair, live with you would affect family dynamics. It might be a wonderful opportunity for everyone to live as a closer family unit, but it will take some adjustment just as any major change in the household would.

It might also be a disaster for all concerned, even if only on a trial basis. If you bring someone under your family roof for care, other members of the family have to continue to live their lives and adhere to their daily routines. Adding an extra person may impose obligations requiring full agreement in advance. Having your brother Sam come to live with you may sound like fun, but if Sam smokes, curses, dresses like a slob, and smells, his fitting in (and your getting used to him being around all the time) is not going to be easy. If Grandma has dementia and follows family members around asking repetitive questions and driving everyone to distraction, the rest of the family may become hostile. Think carefully before choosing this option.

If you are currently a long-distance caregiver and are considering relocating the person you are caring for to your neighborhood or town, think carefully. Although it would be convenient for you to have the person nearby when care is needed, it may not be the best choice. It is important to consider that uprooting someone who is already at risk and relocating him or her far away from a network of friends and ties to a community could be a serious mistake, especially if it will deprive the person of the love, affection, and opportunities the person enjoys for socializing. The old neighborhood friends may prove very helpful when care is needed.

Questions You Need to Ask Before Deciding on a Move

Sometimes, even though everyone loves Mom or Dad, having one of them live in your home is a burden beyond your emotional and physical capability. Whether a parent, sibling, child, relative, or friend is the one needing home care, the following questions must be asked before making a final decision to move someone into your home. Most of these questions would also apply if *you* were moving in with a parent or another person. The relationships will make or break caregiving success.

- What role will the person have in the family? If the person is your parent or grandparent, things will be different from your childhood relationship. Your life and your priorities have changed. They may still see you as a child needing their guidance on decision-making. They may not recognize your changes. Also, parents and family now have different relationships to consider, such as marriages.

- Do prior relationships create home-sharing problems at this stage of your life?

- Will Dad (or you) have to sell or dispose of furnishings and treasures because of limited space?

- How will privacy be provided for you, other family members, and the person needing care?

- How will the new living arrangement work financially?

- How will this affect contributions (in dollars and time) currently being made by other family members?

- How will having a new person with different habits and needs living in the home affect members of your household, your spouse and children?

- What changes need to be made for everyone to accommodate everyone else's habits and needs?

- How will having added responsibilities and obligations for another person alter other facets of your life (personal relationships, work, socializing, etc.)?

- Can you make changes to work and lifestyle without changing your independence in the process?

- Are there other choices?

If a move is necessary, steps can be taken to ease stress for everyone, regardless if the person moves into your home or another housing option or you move into his or her home. Remember:

The new place will never be "home."

- Acknowledge that the new place will never be "home," but that it can be comfortable and tailored to personal comfort and taste.

- Keep the person who is moving as involved as possible in planning the move.

- If furniture, household goods, and family mementos cannot be moved because of limited space, remember that the issue is what can be moved, not what is inheritable (this is not the same as a distribution after the reading of the will). Be sure what is being done follows your loved one's wishes to the greatest degree possible.

- Get an estate appraiser to value the contents of the person's home that need to be disposed of, if a valuation is needed for tax purposes or for a charitable donation. Ask the appraiser for a list of people and companies that purchase households. If items are valuable, consigning them for auction is another alternative.

- Get phone and TV service installed for the person's use ahead of time and have it available on moving day.

- On the day of the move, be prepared to deal with stressful emotions—yours, his, hers, and those of other family members and friends.

If the person is moving into a SNF or ALF or other another environment outside the family home:

- Well before the move, check with staff to determine the best arrival time, personal belongings that can be brought, what to expect during the first few days, and how to make transitioning easier.

- Move a few of the person's personal things into the new place ahead of time, so the space seems more familiar and home-like.

- Facilities use a communal laundry, so mark the person's name on everything.

- If space is limited, focus on making the place feel more personal.

Security/Safety/Condition Check

Whether a private home or facility is being used for care, it is very important that the surrounding grounds, entrance, inside spaces, and other elements of the residence are examined for security and safety hazards and general condition. Following the "Security/Safety/Condition Survey" in this chapter as you look over a residence will result in a more thorough picture of the condition of the property and help you determine whether it is safe and possible space for a person to live securely and healthily, as well as what improvements would be necessary (if feasible).

When evaluating whether any location is the best location for providing needed care, keep in mind that care facilities *are not* and *cannot* be the same as a family home and that family homes, group homes, and care facilities have different uses and purposes, and standards for care and lifestyle may differ. Your ability to make changes in a group home or facility will be limited. However, whether the place is a family home, group home, or a facility, the place in which a loved one lives has to ensure safety, security, and quality of life. It never hurts to ask whether a change is possible.

The place in which a loved one lives has to ensure safety, security, and quality of life.

The Survey shows more than just the obvious—even small things can be serious when someone has a disability, is frail, has simple infirmities, or even the normal limitations of aging.

TIP: In many communities police and fire departments offer an in-home safety inspection program. A department representative will walk through and around the home offering ideas on how to make the home safer and more secure.

 TIP: There is a big difference between maintaining a house in a safe manner and making it usable as a location to deliver care. The process of modifying a home for use by the frail or disabled is much more complicated and comprehensive than childproofing a home for a healthy toddler's curiosity. For example, some changes that you make—adding an outside ramp, for example—may require building permits and compliance with laws and regulations.

 TIP: When considering care at home, you have to consider a variety of elements. For example, if your husband weighs 180 pounds and you weigh 110 pounds, it is more than likely you will have trouble handling his weight, transferring him from wheelchair to bed and back again can pose a physical danger to you both. A Hoyer lift may solve the problem but not if you do not know what it is, where to get it, how to pay for it, and if it won't fit because of a low ceiling. Doorways may be too narrow for the wheelchair and corners too tight to make turns easily. You may need better lighting or a bedside commode—the list goes on and on, and new things will be added over time. You need the Plan to prepare for change.

SECURITY/SAFETY/CONDITION SURVEY

This survey is primarily for a family home. However, it may be used when you tour a group home or facility, in addition to other questions you will have (e.g., number of staff per resident).

Indicate by checking either "yes" or "no" to indicate the accuracy of each statement. If something needs repair, replacement, or rearrangement make a note of what needs to be done.

Is the statement correct?	Yes	No	If the answer is no, describe condition.
Roof and House Exterior/Windows			
The roof is in good condition and requires no repair. Note when installed: _____			
Gutters (if present) are in good condition.			
The siding/bricks/other material is in good condition and needs no repair.			
The painted surfaces are in good condition and require no repainting.			
Windows are equipped with screens, easy to open, and have no cracks or broken panes.			
Windows are in good condition and caulking is secure.			
Electrical Outlets, Electrical and Other Cords, Electrical System			
Electric outlets are at least 6 inches from the floor.			
All appliances are within 27 inches of an outlet.			
Use of extension cords is avoided.			
Electrical and telephone cords are anchored or clear of pathways.			
The electrical system is up to date and has sufficient power to run the house and all appliances.			

Is the statement correct?	Yes	No	If the answer is no, describe condition.
Plumbing and Water Systems			
Sinks and tubs are free of leaks and in good condition.			
The hot water heater is conveniently located.			
The hot water heater is in good condition and easy to maintain.			
Air Conditioning and Heating System			
The air conditioner/heating system is in good condition. Enter date installed: _____			
The system filters are changed monthly.			
Room Arrangements, Furniture, and Appliances			
Window and door locks are secure and in good repair.			
Thermostats are manageable and within easy reach.			
Stairways are free of clutter, well-lit, and in good repair.			
Chairs and sofas are easy to get in and out of.			
The home has a bedroom and full bathroom on the first floor. The washer and dryer are on the same floor as the bedroom.			
Floors are clear of clutter.			
There are no unsecured area rugs or scatter rugs on the floors.			
The flooring in the home is smooth and slip-resistant.			
Carpet has a low pile and a firm pad in good repair and is tacked down.			
Closets and Closet Organization			
Belongings not used are thrown away or donated promptly.			

Is the statement correct?	Yes	No	If the answer is no, describe condition.
Most things in closets are reachable even if the person is sitting.			
Clothing rods are 20 to 44 inches above the floor.			
There is a closet organizing system with drawers and shelves.			
Drawers are no more than 30 inches from the floor.			
The drawers are full-extension and pull out all the way.			
Shelves are no more than 18 inches deep.			
Lower drawers are deep and upper drawers are shallow.			
There are special shoe shelves on the wall.			
In each closet, there is a light with an easy-to-reach switch.			
The closet doors are at least 32 inches wide.			
Laundry Room			
The laundry room is on the first floor.			
The washing machine is front loading.			
All laundry supplies are within easy reach.			
A rolling cart or fold-down shelf is available to use when sorting clothing.			
Kitchen			
Frequently used kitchen items are easy to reach.			
Stove controls are easy to read and operate.			

Is the statement correct?	Yes	No	If the answer is no, describe condition.
Bathrooms			
Grab bars have been installed in the bathroom by the tub, shower, and toilet.			
Bathmats are nonskid.			
Nonskid adhesive strips are on the bottom of the tub or shower.			
A shower seat and handheld showerhead are present.			
Bathroom outlets are GFI outlets.			
Telephones			
Telephones are in the main bedroom and one other room.			
There is at least one cordless phone.			
If the person is to use a cell phone, he or she knows how to use it and is physically able to do so; the charging cord and station are convenient and easy for him or her to use; and he or she carries it in a convenient pouch, purse, or pocket at all times.			
Outdoor Pathways			
A clear path leads from the curb to the house.			
The path slopes gently and is not steep.			
The path is at least 36 inches wide.			
Shrubs are cut back on the side of the path.			
The path is free of berries or leaves.			
The path has no holes in the pavement.			

Is the statement correct?	Yes	No	If the answer is no, describe condition.
The path has a textured surface.			
The path is well-lit.			
Outdoor lights are on motion detectors.			
There is a handrail (if needed) on the front steps.			
Every step has a nonslip surface.			
Ramps (if needed)			
There is a professionally built ramp at the home.			
The ramp complies with all local and state regulations and is ADA compliant.			
The ramp is not steep.			
The ramp is built close to the house.			
There is a landing at the top of the ramp.			
There is a landing at the bottom of the ramp.			
There is a landing in the middle of a long ramp.			
There is a landing each time the ramp changes direction.			
Each landing is 60 inches long and 60 inches wide.			
The ramp is level from side to side.			
The surface isn't slippery when wet.			
There are guardrails to keep users from falling off.			
The guardrails are 18 inches from the ramp floor.			

Is the statement correct?	Yes	No	If the answer is no, describe condition.
There are handrails on both sides of the ramp.			
The handrails are made of sturdy material.			
Handrails extend at least 12 inches beyond the ramp.			
There is a 2-inch edging along the ramp floor.			
There are stairs that can be used by people who do not need a ramp.			
Lighting			
Full use of natural light is made by opening curtains and shades.			
Reading chairs are near a window.			
Windows are clean.			
Incandescent lights are used, and fluorescent lights are avoided.			
The highest wattage bulbs allowed are used for each light fixture.			
Light bulbs change easily.			
Three-way bulbs are in all reading lamps.			
Floor lamps provide direct light where needed.			
All stairways are amply lit.			
There is a light switch at the top and bottom of each staircase.			
Nightlights are used especially between bedrooms and bathrooms.			
Rocker light switches are used throughout the house.			

Is the statement correct?	Yes	No	If the answer is no, describe condition.
Light fixtures inside and outdoors are easy to clean and cleaned frequently.			
Outdoor walkways are well-lit.			
Outside lights turn on automatically.			
Flashlights are handy in the bedroom, kitchen, and living areas.			
A lamp in each room can be turned on using a switch by the door.			
There is an electric outlet on the light switch near each door.			
Household Security System			
The control panels for the security system are within easy reach.			
The following people have access codes: (list)			
Each person has a different code.			
Everyone has the same code.			
The codes are recorded in the following location(s): (list)			
Instructions for calling security are clearly posted near access panels and telephones.			
There is a battery backup for the security system.			
The backup lasts for (enter length of time):			
Smoke Detectors/Alarms/Fire Extinguishers			
A smoke detector is on each floor of the home (including basement).			
There is at least one battery-operated detector.			
There is at least one detector on electric current.			

Is the statement correct?	Yes	No	If the answer is no, describe condition.
Smoke detectors are outside each bedroom.			
Smoke detectors are ceiling mounted.			
Smoke detector batteries are changed at least twice a year. Date last changed: _____			
Smoke alarms are vacuumed once a year.			
Smoke alarms are tested once a month.			
There is a fire extinguisher on each floor.			
There is an extra fire extinguisher in the kitchen.			
Extinguishers are inspected regularly and replaced or recharged as needed.			
Everyone knows how to use a fire extinguisher.			
Doors, building materials, carpeting, etc., are fire resistant.			
Everyone knows what to do when the smoke detector sounds.			
Routes for getting out in an emergency have been planned and practiced, and people know how to remove someone who is disabled.			
In an emergency, windows can be opened to allow escape from or access to rooms. (Note: In a secure facility, windows may have locks or screens that cannot be easily removed; however, staff or several family members should know how to open locks and remove screens.)			
Cleanliness			
The residence is well maintained; corners are as clean as the center of rooms, and it is clear that cleaning is done regularly.			

Additional notes can be entered at the end of your survey.

If you used the survey to review a facility or group home, after you have finished the survey make a list of issues you noted, beginning with safety and cleanliness issues. Discuss your concerns with staff. Keep in mind that a facility or a group home may not be as perfect as you would expect your own home to be. The question is will it provide a safe, secure place where quality of life is assured.

If you used the survey to review a private residence, once you have completed the survey make a summary list of changes that should be made. Look at the cost to make the changes—cost of materials, needed professional support, etc. Look at resources available to make the changes—time, skills of unpaid workers, engineers, general contractors, other needed professional support, permits, inspections, and so forth.

Some things can be done on your own (e.g., remove scatter rugs). For others, you may need to seek a professional. Ask whether the benefit of making the change makes the cost worth the effort. For example, rewiring a house to improve the electrical system is costly.

If resources are limited, prioritize the list based on safety and ease of caregiving.

After considering these factors, you can decide whether modifying the residence is feasible or not. If it is, put plans into place to make it happen. If it is not, put plans into place to make a move.

Hiring a Paid Caregiver

If you are a working caregiver, someone who is taking care of children, a long-distance caregiver, or a primary caregiver who has physical limitations of your own, you may need in-home, paid help. Many situations warrant paid caregiver services to supplement care provided by you and others. This is true when the person needing care

- requires assistance with routine activities of daily living (ADLs), such as bathing, dressing, or toileting;
- requires assistance with moving about and routine household tasks, such as preparing meals, shopping, and housekeeping;

- manages well during the day, but there is concern when he or she is alone at night;

- suffers from early stage dementia or a physical condition that could result in a fall or other injury;

- is physically and mentally capable but socially isolated.

Each situation is unique, and only you and the person who needs care, as well as participating family members, can decide whether paid help is necessary. If help is needed, there are options to consider, as described in other sections of the *Manual*.

And remember, living alone does not have to mean being lonely.

- **Regardless of age, contact with other people is extremely important.** Mom may need social activity (actual human contact) brought into the home. If she manages fairly well on her own, try and locate a volunteer companion who can stop by, stay for an hour, visit, socialize, and leave. These visitors will not be there to do chores or provide hands-on care. (Visitors can monitor whether she continues to function "fairly well" or begins to have increased difficulty that means more help is needed.)

  Living alone does not have to mean being lonely.

- **Trained personnel from a telephone assurance program can call** daily (or once or twice a week) at a set time to see what Mom's doing and perhaps remind her it's time to take medication.

- **Emergency alert systems** are invaluable when an emergency occurs and Mom is alone. She can use her emergency pager (a necklace or a wristband) to signal for help, and a call center attendant will respond immediately.

- You can use **an in-home web cam** ("granny cam") to check in on your child or see how your aunt is doing using your office or home computer. Whether you are a dad at work or a long-distance caregiver, you can even watch to see how in-home aides and paid workers attend and respond to the needs of your loved one. Assure your aunt that using the camera is to ensure her well-being, not to spy on her.

- If your sister Claire cannot prepare her own meals because of her Parkinson's disease, try **having meals delivered** to her home. She may be eligible to participate in the local meal delivery program, and the volunteer or paid delivery person who delivers hot meals can offer a few moments of socialization and check to make sure Claire is okay.

- Many grocery stores have **prepackaged fresh meals**. You or a paid shopper can buy for the week and freeze them along with other groceries to either reduce dependency on meal services or even provide all meals.

- Ask **a neighbor to drop in** occasionally to share a meal or a snack and spend a little time.

- For variety or in a pinch, have **local restaurants deliver** cooked meals. Keep menus handy for your use (and the use of your loved one) make sure restaurant names and phone numbers are clearly visible. You can order by credit card (tip included) and have a hot meal at the front door. Call Granddad and tell him, "Food is on the way, and it is paid for already," so he will not be taken advantage of by double billing.

- If you are a long-distance caregiver, arrange in advance for **local help**—a GCM or home care agency—who can step in to handle things before you get there.

All of these activities will not only ensure your loved one's safety and well-being but can offer a variety of social contact where it is needed. Whether you live on the next block, in the next county, or across the country, a combination of services will ensure your loved one has daily human contact.

Fundamentals of Hiring and Managing In-Home Care Services

As care needs and home assistance escalates, you may require someone to provide care several hours each day. You should have anticipated this need as part of the planning process. If the need is a surprise, the process of hiring and managing in-home care services will be the same. There are only two options for hiring—you contact a reputable home healthcare agency and pay them to provide qualified in-home staff or you hire someone independently.

Before Hiring

Whether you hire help through an agency or directly, you need to do the following before you hire:

- **Check the Plan.** Which family members can help (contribute time or money) with care?

- Check with Uncle Paul's physician to make sure the **clinical skills required** to provide quality care that you outlined in the Plan are still accurate.

- Check the Plan to make sure it still accurately represents how your loved one handles self-care tasks. *Basic* self-care tasks include bathing, walking, eating, selecting clothes, and grooming (called Activities of Daily Living or ADLs by professionals), and more *complex* self-care tasks include managing finances, preparing meals, managing public transportation, and managing medication (called Instrumental Activities of Daily Living or IADLs by professionals).

- Prepare a **list of duties/responsibilities** to be performed by the person who is hired.

- Develop a **personality profile** of your loved one and consider what the employee needs to be prepared for when working with him or her.

- **Review insurance coverage** so you know what the insurer covers, how to start services, and how reimbursement is handled.

- **Research the costs of care** and the differences when you hire through an agency or hire privately.

Time may be tight, but you will greatly benefit from an organized approach.

Use the checklist on the following pages to prepare a list of duties to be performed, and add duties to it if you know they need to be done but do not see them on this list.

DUTIES TO BE PERFORMED

This checklist will help you define an in-home helper's scope of responsibility and the frequency and length of required services. Indicate which tasks need to be performed. Specify how often and when each duty is to be performed.

Duty	How Often	When
FOOD AND NUTRITION		
Shop for groceries		
Plan for special diet		
Prepare breakfast		
Prepare lunch		
Prepare dinner		
Prepare snacks		
Feed by hand		
Assist with eating		
Encourage to eat		
DRESSING		
Select clothing		
Assist with dressing		
Assist with undressing		

Duty	How Often	When
PERSONAL HYGIENE		
Provide a tub bath		
Assist with showering		
Brush teeth		
Clean dentures		
Shampoo hair		
Brush/comb hair		
Shave		
Clean eyeglasses		
Assist with hearing aid		
Assist with toileting		
HOUSEHOLD CHORES		
Change bed		
Clean bathroom		
Clean kitchen		
Dust		
Empty trash		

Duty	How Often	When
Do general household shopping		
Make bed		
Vacuum		
Wash floors		
Wash/dry dishes		
Iron/fold clothes		
Do home maintenance		
Do yardwork		
ROUTINE TASKS		
Use phone		
Pay bills		
Do banking		
Support socialization		
Read		
Serve as a companion		
Motivate		

Duty	How Often	When
TRANSPORTATION		
Assist on and off provided transportation		
Drive patient's/family's car (If this is required, be sure auto insurance will cover the paid helper driving the car.)		
Drive own car (If this is required, the paid helper's auto insurance will need to cover him or her driving for business purposes; ask for documentation.)		
Drive to and from doctor		
Drive to and from shopping		
Drive to and from social outings		
HEALTHCARE DUTIES		
Prepare medications (The helper may have to be specially licensed to do this.)		
Remind to take medications		
Assist with exercises		
Encourage exercise		
Assist with chair to bed transferring, bed to chair, etc.		
Change dressings		
Manage incontinence		
Assist with mental stimulation exercises		

Duty	How Often	When
OTHER (list specific additional tasks)		

How Do You Match Personalities?

Perfection is rarely found, but compatibility and the potential employee's ability to handle the job are critical. Once you have outlined the duties and the hours, consider personality. If Mom requires twenty-four-hour attention or suffers from dementia, wandering, or paranoia, you may not be able to find even one individual who can adjust to her needs, and that may eliminate the in-home option. Having two or more aides, if affordable, may still make it possible to use paid help at home.

Once you have outlined the duties of the position, talk to family members or professionals who understand home care to confirm that your hiring expectations are reasonable. Sometimes, in-home help is not the solution when the demands of care will combine with difficult personality or behavioral issues.

Use the Personality Compatibility Checklist on the next page to find good matches. While there is no guarantee of success, considering the personality traits of your demanding wife and of a potential paid caregiver makes success more likely.

PERSONALITY COMPATIBILITY CHECKLIST

If the person needing care has one or more of the personality traits listed below, it is important to consider how that trait will affect the relationship with the paid caregiver.

Organized	Disorganized
Used to being in charge	Used to being told what to do
Flexible	Set in his or her ways
Smoker	Nonsmoker
Assertive	Passive
Outgoing/social	Shy

In addition, consider whether there are concerns as follows:

- Ethnic, language, and cultural differences that could be communication barriers.
- Age differences—too young or too old.
- Tolerance and appreciation for your loved one's interests.

How Many People Do You Really Need?

Once you have determined the duties and schedule of the paid caregiver, ask yourself whether one person is enough. Be realistic. One person can handle a few hours a day, every day, or once or twice a week, but perhaps around-the-clock help is needed. Do you need help only when you are at work, only on weekends, a couple of nights a week, every night?

A burned-out, paid caregiver is no better than a burned-out, unpaid family caregiver.

Most states limit work hours for paid caregivers. Also, a "live-in" provider needs a break like everyone else and usually works 5.5 days with 1.5 days off. Schedules vary, but time off is an important element in hiring. A burned-out, paid caregiver is no better than a burned-out, unpaid family caregiver.

What about Benefits?

Agencies who hire their own staff for placement in your home typically pay all required taxes and Worker's Compensation for employees. However, if the agency is actually a registry (a listing of available workers who are not employees of the agency but who use the agency as a source of referrals for getting private work), the agency typically does not pay benefits. Be very clear whose paying before accepting the employee.

If you are the employer, you are responsible for the employer's portion of Social Security (FICA), Federal Unemployment Tax (FUTA), state unemployment tax, and State Worker's Compensation contributions. For details contact local state employment and Social Security offices or call your accountant or a CPA. Remember, employees deserve similar considerations of reasonable schedules, breaks, and time off that you would expect if hired for the job.

Everyone dreams about finding that one wonderful helper who moves in and becomes another family member. Sometimes it occurs and a dedicated and loyal helper is found. However, manage your expectations—that person may never be found, or you may have to go through a number of employees before you find the right one.

The Job Description

If home care seems best, a clear job description with detailed performance expectations creates a specific understanding for the potential worker. Descriptions should include:

- Hours of work
- Specific duties
- Special abilities needed (driving, lifting, etc.)
- Desirable personality traits
- Language spoken
- Days off and work breaks
- Hourly/daily/weekly rate

- License or certification required. Check with the state board that oversees healthcare to see what is required. **Note:** Being a private employee does not mean the person is exempted from having a license. For example, in your state it is likely illegal for someone without a license to give medication.

Hiring Potential Employees Without an Agency

Before using a paid want ad, there are alternatives that may be more successful:

- **Be cautious about the information you include when you make announcements or post notices**. What you say and where you say it may alert unscrupulous people that your loved one is in a vulnerable situation. Do not give the address where care will be provided. Do not use your loved one's name or phone number. Would Aunt Gracie give out personal information if a stranger calls? Use your first name and the number of a phone you will answer.

- **Ask around.** Talk to coworkers, neighbors, and friends to see if they have needed paid caregivers in the past. If a particular name comes up often, take action. Find out his or her availability for work; if not, ask if he or she knows someone who is available.

- **Post notices** in local pharmacies or neighborhood supermarkets. Try church or temple bulletins and newsletters. Try organizations you or Dad belong to (or used to belong to).

- If a special set of skills or license/certification is required, **say so in any advertisement or announcement**.

- If you run a want ad in the newspaper or online, try to **avoid abbreviating words**; abbreviations can be confusing. You do not have to print the entire job description, but do include statements like "required to prepare meals, assist with daily needs, drive own car on errands." Ads may be expensive, but the clearer you are in stating needs, the fewer inappropriate responses you will receive.

Screening Callers

Be ready for calls and to ask the right questions. The initial contact is to find out about the person calling. If a caller is experienced and understands what may be required, you should not have to go into much detail.

To better screen the caller, create a script (write down the questions). This will ensure you will tell everyone the same things and get the same information from them. For example:

Thank you for responding to the ad.

Where did you see the ad?

What are your full name, address, and telephone number?

Why are you interested in the job?

What experience do you have in this kind of work?

Are you currently employed?

Why do you want to leave your present position?

What days and times are you available to work?

What salary and benefits do you expect?

Ask questions vital to personal preferences, such as the following:

Do you have a car and a valid drivers license?

Do you smoke?

How do you feel about pets?

Are you comfortable cooking special dietary meals?

Do you cook foods with strong odors?

Restate important requirements, such as the following:

The tasks you are to perform require you to be licensed by the state (or certification). Do you have a current license?

I must inform you that I will be checking references and conducting a thorough background check, including a criminal background check, before hiring anyone.

If You Are Interested in Setting Up an Interview

Ask: *When can you meet me here for an interview?*

Set a time: *Okay, we will meet at _____ o'clock on [day, date] at my Dad's house. The address is _____.*

Tell him or her: *Please bring a copy of your resume, references, and certification with you.*

Close by saying: *I look forward to seeing you on [date] at [time].*

Pay attention to your gut instinct. If a person does not "feel" right to you, he or she probably is not the right person to provide care.

Not Interested?

Tell him or her: *Thank you for calling. I have just begun to interview people by phone. I will call if I am interested in having a face-to-face interview.*

Unless a candidate seems totally unsuitable, do not close the door entirely. Experienced, in-home workers are rare. Having a list of potential workers for short-term emergency coverage is also very helpful.

Scheduling and Conducting the Face-to-Face Interview

When you schedule face-to-face interviews, do not schedule them too closely together. Allow plenty of time to ask questions, explain needs, and respond to questions.

As you did when you were screening, write down questions in advance so everyone provides similar information, but do not limit questions to what is written. Think about what the person being interviewed is saying and make sure you understand.

As the potential employer you have a right to ask reasonable questions. The people you interview will provide information that needs to be verified. You also need to be observant about attitudes and behavior. Consider the following:

- **Think carefully about where to hold the initial interview.** You may want to conduct the first part of the interview away from the house where care will be provided to avoid compromising the safety and security of the person needing care (or the security of your own home). If the first part of the interview goes well, you can always schedule a "part two" in the home so your loved one can meet the potential employee and see how they get along before making an offer.

- If you are interviewing several people, **ask permission to take their pictures using your cell phone or camera** to keep track of everyone. Pictures in a cell phone gallery are typically identified by date and time or by a photo number—make a note on each person's resume indicating which picture is his or hers. (Use the labels created for each picture on your cell phone or camera to identify each one accurately.) Be sensitive to the fact that some people do not like their picture to be taken; that does not mean something is wrong, but they may have their own concerns about privacy.

- **Was the candidate on time?** If not, why not? Timeliness is very important in providing in-home care. You are relying on the person you hire to be on time. Ask whether he or she drove to the interview, were driven by someone else, or took public transportation.

- **Did the candidate bring a resume, references, and copies of his or her license** or certification if needed?

- Ask whether the candidate is **working more than one job**. A person working multiple jobs may have difficulty getting from one job to another on time or may not be flexible enough to handle scheduling needs.

- **Ask for details on past experience**, and ask questions that give a sense of the person's ability to respond to Mom's needs.

- **Ask "what if" questions**: "What if Dad won't eat?"; "What if Mom gets angry and orders you to leave?"; "What if Grandpa falls getting out of his wheelchair?"; "What if there's a major emergency like a stroke?"; "What if your car breaks down and you can't get to work?"

- Pay attention to **nonverbal details**, such as personal grooming, personality traits, and how the person responds in the interview. Is the candidate polite and courteous with a positive attitude? Are answers openly offered? Does the candidate make eye contact or stare at the floor and fidget? The latter are characteristics typical of a person uncomfortable with interviews or with telling the full truth.

- Consider how **personalities will mesh**.

- Ask about the applicant's **physical health**.

- Introduce Mom and observe the way she and the candidate respond to each other. If having paid help is an issue for Mom, expect to see her react about that now. How did the prospective employee respond to the resistance?
- Remind the person that you will be **checking references and conducting a background check**.
- **Make notes** so you don't forget your observations.

After the Interview

- **Review your notes and weigh all information**. Chances are no interviewee will meet every qualification. However, keep the most critical keys to quality care in mind. Prioritize qualifications by their importance; for example, personality compatibility is more important than how they get to work.
- **Consider issues of concern that arose during the interview.** If the candidate claimed care experience but presented no references, you need to be concerned.
- **Always check references.** No matter how likable the applicant or how badly help is needed, thoroughly check references. You need to know about trustworthiness, adaptability, and performance under stress. Briefly describe your expectations. Ask former employers if they think the applicant can handle the job.
- **Conduct a background check.** The information obtained from a criminal background check will make a major difference in whether you decide to hire the person. A person with a criminal background that includes assault, for example, is not a good candidate to care for your frail Aunt. Not all states allow a criminal background check, but you can contact local police to see how to conduct one. In some states, there are legally licensed businesses that will do a background check for a fee. A Level II check is one that searches throughout the entire country for a person's record. A name and social security number is all that's required, along with a fee. (By law, some states require that anyone, whether paid or unpaid, related or unrelated, who has contact with a person needing care undergo a background check.)

After Making Your Choice

The extra work of a thorough interview and background check saves the misery, cost, and danger created by minimal verification. Quality help is essential to providing quality care.

Remember, the goal of the Plan is your peace of mind and ensuring the safety and quality of life of your loved one. You did your homework and made the wisest choice you could based on the information and the circumstances your investigation revealed.

Once your selection is made, make your offer, and if accepted, create a **written employment contract**. Have a basic contract prepared in advance (see below). Blank contract forms can be found in most office supply stores; if you use one, be careful filling in the details and attach your schedule of duties.

On the first day of work, go over the contact with the employee and have him or her provide any missing information. Either two copies of the contract should be signed (one for you and one for the employee), or you should be prepared to make a copy of the signed document for the employee. You keep the original. Give the employee the copy to take home.

After signing the agreement, the employee should complete and sign a W-9 form. Remember: As an employer, you need to pay and report income and taxes for this employee. Also, if you are able to claim a tax deduction or need to document an expense for insurance purposes, such records are essential.

Employment Contract

To ensure a complete understanding of the work expected, prepare a written description of what is required, confirming details of required services. This contract should list at least the following items.

- **Employer and employee name:** For example: "Employment Contract between (insert name of employer) and (insert name of employee) . . . "
- **Employee's Social Security number**
- **Scheduled hours** of work
- **Pay rate:** dollars per hour

- **Pay schedule:** How often and in what form (cash, check).

- **Benefits as applicable:** Time off and schedule for time off, reimbursement for the employee using his or her car (if that is required), meals you provide, sleeping quarters if the person is a live-in employee, etc.

- **Duties** (be specific): Copy the list you prepared earlier in this section or attach a copy to the contract and note, "Duties are specified in the attached list" or something similar.

- **Telephone use:** Define when and how the employee may use his or her cell phone or the house phone when on duty. Phone use should be limited to calls to you to report on what is going on, calls necessary to performing his or her duties (e.g., confirming medical transportation arrival times), and no personal calls except in an emergency (e.g., child's illness). The rules should apply even when Mom is sleeping.

- **Termination statement warning:** If the employer or the family caregiver provides feedback to the employee that a work habit (e.g., tardiness) or behavior (list critical actions, such as leaving the person needing care alone) must be changed and the habit or behavior is not remedied after two weeks' notice, the employee will be terminated.

- **Immediate termination** for theft, failure to perform assigned duties, unacceptable or dangerous behavior affecting Uncle Ed.

- **Acknowledgment by employee:** Use language such as, "I understand my written duties and the terms set out in this agreement and agree to perform them to the best of my ability."

- **Employee Signature**

- **Date Signed**

- **Employer's Signature**

Retaining the Employee

Once you find an employee and the contract is signed, the next goal is to make sure the employee stays on the job.

- **Allow for an adjustment period.** Make sure the person knows you are available and how to reach you during the scheduled work hours. Keep checking in and let him or her know everyone wants things to work.

- **Do not assume** the employee can step right into the job simply because he or she has prior experience. Your new hire may have a great deal of experience but does not yet have any working relationship with Dad. Your support and guidance during the early weeks is important. Working through things together can be the difference between keeping and losing a good worker.

- Provide the person with **as much information as possible** about your loved one, work requirements, the household, and so on. For example, if Dad is likely to try and do everything himself or not ask for help—even when in jeopardy of falling—explain that in advance. Show the helper where things are in the home—linens, cleaning supplies, medications, and the like. We all expect our new hire to know where we keep things and how we like things done, but that is not a realistic expectation.

- If a worker is required to drive (whether he or she uses his or her car or your family car) or do shopping, **discuss how gas will be reimbursed, groceries paid for, etc.** The worker may have a tight budget that does not allow him or her to pay. A system may have to be put into place for providing payment funds in advance or immediate reimbursement. Dealing upfront with these items is professional and sets a professional standard.

- **Openly discuss cancellations and absences.** Reliability is not negotiable, but things happen. Discuss and agree on how to handle these emergencies and have a backup plan. For example, does the worker have experienced and reliable relative or friend who could cover an absence? If so, ask to meet the person. It is advisable to ask for references, as well as to consider doing a background check.

- **Discuss the importance of setting house rules regarding telephone use, visitors, smoking, music, routines for care of your loved one**. The use of any illegal substance must be cause for immediate termination. Review meal time and bed time routines, bathing (bath vs. shower), special ways to communicate if communicating with Mom is difficult, etc.

- If the worker is expected to **give medicine**, make sure all instructions are clear. Provide detailed instructions, preferably in writing. Prepare a list of medications, dosages, schedule for taking each dose, and other specific details. It is useful to state things like, "Give two orange pills at 8:00 a.m. and one purple pill with food no later than 1:00 p.m.; give no liquids after 9:00 p.m." Perhaps you need to load a pill box (one that shows days or days and times of day). Instruct the worker to observe Uncle Hal taking and swallowing his pills.

- **Watch for warning signs of possible problems**. Verify that medications are being taking by counting pills and noting use of liquids. Check the mileage on the car (take a picture of the odometer). Take pictures of the car before the worker starts using it (inside and out) and examine the car periodically to make sure it is in the same condition it was when he or she began to drive it. Check work to insure it is being done as agreed. Monitor the use of supplies and money: Are there dramatic increases in money spent for groceries and household expenses? Does Mom express dissatisfaction or has she changed the way she talks about the person? Does your daughter show fear of the person? Is there a pattern of increasing employee absences or later arrivals? Keep an eye on small valuables and jewelry (even jewelry your loved one always wears).

- **Are you concerned you are not getting the whole picture when you ask** the employee for information? Are you concerned the employee does not bring issues that might be of concern to your attention without being asked? If so, that is *very* problematic. Be sure communication is clear and thorough on both sides. Make sure the person understands that you expect to be told about what is going on. Encourage the person to be open, even when something has happened that could be seen as "bad." Make sure the person knows that YOU know accidents are accidents and sometimes cannot be prevented, even by the most careful caregiver (paid or unpaid). Provide a bound notebook and instruct the employee to write down what happens each day while caring for your loved one (e.g., behavior that caused concern, activities he or she engaged in), supplies that are running low and should be purchased, and other issues that can easily be forgotten unless written down. At the end of the day, add your own comments about, for example, how a behavior could have been handled, when supplies will be purchased, an activity that the paid helper could help with, and so on. These daily notes can remind an employee about what is expected without being confrontational and also can serve as a diary of interaction that can help you assess the paid helper's performance.

- If a paid caregiver **behaves in a manner causing you or Dad concern**, take immediate action. Meet with the caregiver and describe the behavior in question. Be specific, give details, and set a time frame for change. Remind the employee of the contract and the consequences for failure to change. Be prepared to enforce and live with the consequences of no change.

- Finally, make it clear to the employee that **you are counting on him or her** as a professional to give you valuable insight about Dad and noticeable changes in health or behavior. Acknowledge that caring can be difficult work and demonstrate respect the employee's professionalism. Tell him or her you are available to work through difficult situations or job frustrations. In sum, work to build a solid relationship based on mutual trust and respect.

Ask yourself, "What makes me feel good about my job?" Is it your employer's trust in you with real responsibility? Does he or she seek your ideas and opinions and make you feel like a team player? Do you perform your job in a pleasant and safe environment? Is your pay fair? Your employee deserves no less consideration.

TIP: From an employer's perspective, most jobs in the workplace do not demand the intensity of one-on-one home care. Care for hours at a time with potential age, culture, and gender barriers is tough. In a hospital, SNF, ALF, or rehab there are strong internal rules of behavior and a hierarchy of people enforcing them. Leaving someone in charge of Mom at home or anywhere requires your patience and faith. Whenever your gut says something is not right, follow your instincts!

TIP: Hiring is a process like any other process in the Plan. Use the steps outlined in this chapter unless your day job is hiring and firing. Do not be afraid to say, "This is not working" and terminate the relationship as of a specific date, if not immediately. It is enough of a burden that you bear responsibility for Mom, but worrying about who is in the house with her is not productive for creating and maintaining your peace of mind.

USING IN-HOME CARE FROM A HOME HEALTHCARE AGENCY

Home healthcare agencies are everywhere. All agencies provide individuals but have different hiring practices. Check an agency as if it were a person you are independently hiring.

Agency Quality of Care

- Obtain references; check licenses.

- Does the agency provide state-funded program services funded, for example, by Child and Family Welfare, Community Care for the Elderly, or Medicaid Waiver? If so, the agency must meet certain basic standards.

- Ask the agency for copies of any monitoring done, copies of licenses, and so forth, and then double check. Has the agency been written up for any violations during monitoring? What kind and were they critical to care delivery? For example, if an agency was written up for using an employee to give medications when the employee was not licensed to do so, that is an important violation. If the agency was written up for filing a required state report ten days late, that may not be important to actual care delivery.

Agency Terms of Service and Work

- **Is the agency a direct employer** (i.e., they hire hourly employees and pay their wages, taxes, etc.) **or a registry** (i.e., they keep a list of individuals who appear to have the credentials to fill job requirements)? Are the workers employees or independent contractors?

- How does the agency select an employee? **What selection criteria are used**?

- Does the agency conduct employment reference and criminal background checks? (Never bring a worker into your home that has not had a criminal background check!)

- Who carries the **liability** insurance, the agency or the employee?

- Pricing: hourly, daily, weekly?

- Billing period: frequency, day of the month, etc.

- Forms of payment accepted.

- Can you **prescreen candidates**?

- How do you **change workers or schedules**?

- What **lead-time is needed to make changes**?

- **Review the agency contract carefully before you sign.** If unsure of the terms, get professional advice.

- **Do not automatically assume any agency is reliable, careful, and honest.** Do your homework and be vigilant.

- Once you choose an agency, **provide the agency with the same written information** about your requirements that you would provide if you were hiring an employee yourself. Describe Mom's care needs and personality, hours of services required, etc. Explain exactly what you expect.

- Once an agency employee is placed in the home, **drop in unannounced** to see how things are going. Do it more than once and on a random schedule. Provide feedback to the employee and share any concerns you have with the employee and with the agency.

- If you are able to **interview an agency employee** before he or she comes into your home, you should ask many of the same questions you would ask if you were hiring someone on your own. Ask about experience, the person's understanding of what will be required of him or her, and other questions that have to do with the person providing the services you require. Observe the person's ability to communicate, level of professionalism, attitudes toward the person needing care, and so forth. If you do not think the employee is right, discuss this with the agency manager.

Complaints

People who are resistant to having someone in the home to provide care have ways of showing their resistance. They may argue with you, be rude to the home care provider, complain all the time, refuse to cooperate, and so on. No matter their age or their condition, people who do not want to cooperate can create a difficult working environment for the in-home worker and for you. However, it is not always the case that those complaints are unfounded.

If Dad complains, pay close attention. He may only be expressing personal frustration or unhappiness with his need for care, but his complaints may also be accurate.

Carefully monitor what is said and what you see. If the complaint is, "I get too little to eat," then monitor food use. If it is, "I am not being bathed," check for wet soap and towels. If he says he is being "yelled at," ask a neighbor about hearing a loud voice. Better yet, place a voice-activated recorder in the home so you can hear what occurs. If you are suspicious or just want to be cautious, use a "nanny cam." Make unexpected visits. Do not assume that Dad is just being annoying or resistant.

Take special care when the paid care provider does not communicate with you openly or respond to questions you ask. If communication is an issue, it may not be the only issue.

Remember that not everyone is loving and kind. Some employees are unhappy, and providing home care creates opportunities to exercise their bad habits and express their frustrations. If Mom complains or shows signs of physical or emotional abuse, take immediate action. Err on the side of caution. Be practical, as well as alert. With some disease and conditions and in the case of thin skin in the elderly, skin tears and bruising are unavoidable occurrences, but they should not occur every few days.

Watch for behavioral changes. Do not ignore signs such as increased depression, avoidance of the person providing care, or outright expressions of fear.

It is far better to be cautious and intervene than to fail to intervene out of fear of being wrong or fear of losing help. If you think there is a problem, immediately remove the worker from the house and contact the agency and/or social service authorities.

YOUR ROLE WHEN SOMEONE ELSE GIVES CARE

It is likely you will need to entrust at least a part of your caregiving to others, and if you are a long-distance caregiver, the probability increases to certainty. Whether with a paid helper, sharing care with family members or other volunteers, or relying on care in an institutional setting, your role as primary caregiver includes monitoring care provided by others. Combined with careful research and selection, the best way to monitor is by visiting the care location during the day while care is being given.

Make Home Visits Count

Regardless of the care setting, each time you visit carefully observe how things are going. Even if you just dropped in to your house during a lunch hour, you can ask the same questions. How is your son Chuck's appetite? Is your wife socializing with friends and neighbors? Is Harry getting enough exercise? Is the environment clean, comfortable, restful, welcoming, safe? Is the care provider calm, organized, empathetic, compassionate, and well prepared for the task?

Every visit should not be an investigation. Use the time to talk and share family and life events. It is important that your sister continues to feel connected to family and friends.

If there are noticeable changes in physical or mental status, talk to your brother's physician or other healthcare professionals about your concerns. If additional help or a change in lifestyle seems indicated, talk it over with your brother (if that is feasible) and enlist his cooperation in finding solutions.

Long Distance Visits

If you live at a distance, use each visit to check in with close neighbors and friends. Ask them how Aunt Sue is managing when you or the worker are not there. Ask if they have any cause for concern. Express appreciation for their help and friendship toward Sue.

Ask for and accept help from others. Allow friends and family to reaffirm their shared friendship with Sue, but be careful not to impose. Stay in touch after returning home and thank them again.

Before leaving, review emergency plans with Aunt Sue and anyone else (neighbor or friend) who might be involved if a crisis occurs. Make it clear that due to distance, you need to rely on them and the emergency plan until you get there.

If you're far away and visits are infrequent, do things to add to the quality of life:

- Have family members schedule **weekly phone calls**. Mix it up and do not have them all call at the same time.

- Send news articles and photos of interest to Aunt Sue. Send them by mail (many people still love to get REAL letters). Use email (if she knows how to use a computer). Give her an easy-to-use fax machine, set it up for her, and show her how to receive and send faxes. (Some stores who sell equipment will also send someone to do this if you ask). Have each niece and nephew send her a daily "child-a-gram" or rotate sending a letter each week.

- Try **new equipment** (a DVD player, an iPod). Aunt Sue's hearing may be better with an iPod and ear buds, and she can more easily enjoy recordings or audio books.

- Have **younger children** create drawings; **older ones** can write a note or send a card.

- Give Aunt Sue a **long distance calling card** and encourage her to call.

- **Call often**. Share news of friends, work, and other activities. Even if Aunt Sue never met the folks being discussed, she will appreciate you sharing your life.

- Ask Aunt Sue for her **advice and opinions**.

ADVOCATE FOR A PERSON LIVING AWAY FROM HOME
Being an Advocate Is Serious Business

When someone moves into an ALF or SNF, that person's "roof" changes, but your responsibility does not end. While free of daily, hands-on assistance, you need to monitor your loved one's care and possibly make adjustments to his or her new circumstances.

Family caregivers become advocates when home is no longer the setting. Being an advocate means staying on top of things, including changes in medication, doctor visits, socialization schedules, eating habits, exercise, and all the things you would check on if your husband were living at home. It is particularly important to make sure his medical file contains instructions to notify you immediately prior to any planned medical care outside the facility (e.g., tests, procedures) and of any changes in his medication (type, dosages, frequency) and who ordered the care or medication changes and why. Do not be afraid to push until you get the complete answer. Never be satisfied with incomplete explanations like, "The doctor said to."

> **Family caregivers become advocates when home is no longer the setting.**

Make Visits Count When Home Is Away from Home

When a person you are caring for relocates to a facility setting, your initial visits may be filled with helping him or her settle in and meeting staff. Getting you and your loved one acclimated to the new setting is critical. Eventually, you may find less to do. Visits may seem monotonous and boring for both of you. However, the fact that most practical care is provided by others affords you and your loved one opportunities to spend quality time together.

Here are some ideas to make visits pleasant and positive for you both:

- **Plan the visit before going**. If possible, let Mom know you have something special planned to look forward to.

- **Get there on time.** If the plan is to get out or do something with other residents, let the staff know in advance.

- **Bring along conversation starters**: photos, crafts, and drawings from the grandchildren; a keepsake you'd like to know more about; or an article in the local newspaper.

- If appropriate, **bring a project to share**. Update photo albums, clip coupons, or bring a mail order catalog to shop for needed clothing or gifts. If you have a very well-behaved pet, ask if it can visit. It will be beneficial for your mom and for others.

- If you are visiting a child, bring along one of the stuffed animals she likes or a new hand-held computer game to play, or just plan on taking a walk outside to look at the plants, trees, and birds. Think about what the child likes to do and is able to do, considering his or her condition, and plan accordingly. Better yet, if the child knows the rules about what he or she can do, ask the child!

- **Do you have a special talent**, such as playing the piano or singing? Occasionally you might offer to entertain everyone.

- **Check the facilities' activity schedule.** Mark the calendar with activities your friend might enjoy. Plan to attend some events together.

- If possible, **take your sister for a drive or lunch** or to attend a family gathering. Even if she cannot leave the facility, at least take a walk. Having a change of scenery is important.

- **Small pleasures count**: getting a manicure or a shampoo, watching a favorite movie on a portable DVD player, watching a favorite program or sporting events on TV, or listening to music. Repot plants Cousin Ann has received, or, if she is capable, help her do it. Play a favorite card or board game.

- **Involve your wife in planning** for major family events, weddings, or a new baby. Let her share gift ideas and ask her for other suggestions.

- Some visits should **focus on monitoring quality of care, room cleanliness, and services.** Observe staff attitude. Are they welcoming and friendly? Do your questions seem like an interruption, rather than necessary?

- **Check food quality**. Share a meal. Does Aunt Edith eat in a dining room or alone in her room? In the dining room, what are other people at the table like? Are they compatible? How's the service? Are special food needs taken into consideration? If Dad needs help eating, is there available staff to assist? If Mom can eat unassisted, but with some effort, is she given easy-to-manage foods? Are meals nutritious and balanced? Is food appetizing and attractively served?

- **Attend and observe scheduled activities**. Does staff encourage Dad's participation? Is Dad expected to keep track of events and show up if interested? Focus on Dad's reaction to the activity: too frustrating, too juvenile, too patronizing? Does he get real pleasure if only for the moment?

- **Check housekeeping practices.** Perform a white-glove test. Check Mom's room and the building's public areas.

- **Work with staff.** Allow time each visit to get the staff's perspective. Discuss concerns or complaints regarding care. When you next visit, check to see whether promised changes were made. Do not expect miracles. Facilities house a number of people; conditions and amenities will never be the same as those at home.

- **Try and attend the monthly care planning meeting**, during which medical staff, social staff, and others on the care team discuss your loved one's progress and needs. If you cannot attend in person, attend by conference call. If you cannot participate at all, obtain the written meeting report and discuss any items of concern with staff on your next visit or in a phone call. If staff does not welcome you at the meeting, that may be a concern; why would they consider you, the primary family caregiver, an intruder?

When you make regular calls and visits, you are ensuring that your loved one receives better care. Staff will notice your interest and that you are monitoring care.

TIP: There are times when the squeaky wheel gets the grease—you make a request or note a problem, and a change is made. When that happens, always say, "Thank you." Even if what is done was supposed to be part of the service provided, remember that staff is busy and you should appreciate their taking the time to make adjustments. Believe it or not, there are times when fifteen people ask to go to the bathroom simultaneously when there are only ten staff members available to respond, and at the same time, staff is trying to follow normal routines (such as administering medication) and responding to vital care emergencies.

TIP: Say thanks with bakery goods or doughnuts left at the nursing station or in the staff lounge. Give a birthday card to the person who spends the most time with your loved one. Even if every staff member is on a diet and no one wants to admit their age, your gesture of care and concern will be appreciated and remembered. Remember that staff deals with Aunt Effie twenty-four hours a day and seven days per week and care will not be delivered in the same way in a 150-bed facility that you are accustomed to providing care or seeing her care delivered at home. Keep cool, know what you want, say it politely, and put it in writing. After you leave, they still have a facility to run.

9.

Someone Else Deserves Care—You!

Up to this point, a great deal has been said about ways to handle caregiving—steps to take, options you may have, handling people you have to deal with, and so on. But the *Manual* began with a dedication to you, as an individual family caregiver. Now, it is time to talk about the one aspect of care planning that even well-organized family caregivers often overlook and that is typically not covered in the most meticulous plan: the steps you can take to provide *you* with care and ensure *your* quality of life.

Many things go unnoticed until they do not get done or get done poorly. Family caregiving is one of those things. It is hard to explain the challenges of family caregiving, the necessary and unending attention to details, and the frustrations when needed services cannot be found. Add to the burden the fact that your wife, who is in desperate need of care, refuses to cooperate or family members are oblivious and uncaring about the sacrifices you make.

If you are not careful, family caregiving can consume you. Almost unconsciously, you give up bits and pieces of your life until your life becomes only about family caregiving.

Age differences and your relationship with the person you are caring for will impact the caregiving process. Caring for Grandma is very different than caring for your child. Parents and children build history together, learn each other's ways, and test one another as their relationship grows. When you are caring for Mom or Grandpa, the history of the relationship between the two of you has already been written. Things shared in the past affect everything shared in the present. When a friend serves as a family caregiver for a friend, the nature of that friendship may be tested. Family caregiving tests every relationship.

When someone is chronically ill, frail, very young, or aged, what may happen is unpredictable. There may be periods of remarkable improvement when less help is needed and then periods when more help than ever before is needed. The roller-coaster effect amplifies the stress of family caregiving.

Before Taking Action, Take a Moment

Because most people do little planning for a care crisis, the need for care is nearly always accompanied by an element of drama, thoughts like, *What can I do now?* and *How do I do this?* They may feel the need to take immediate action because a loved one is in emotional distress or someone from outside the family is pressing for a decision. Prepared family caregivers with their Plans in hand have a triple advantage:

- A plan for steps that can be taken and who can help
- Accessibility to predetermined options for care and ways to pay for it
- Knowledge of how to define the issue and implement solutions

The Plan's purpose is to make the "job" transition from family member or friend to family caregiver easier.

Be Prepared for Changes in Your Life

As you make arrangements for Dad's care, do not neglect yourself. Your role is not to be a "sacrifice" on the family caregiving altar. Whether the need starts small and grows, or starts large and grows larger, if you do not take care of you, how can you expect to provide for Dad's care?

Stress management pays big dividends. Know your limitations, set achievable goals, and remind yourself you are doing the best you can. You do not get credit for being a martyr in family caregiving. **THERE ARE NO MARTYRS IN FAMILY CAREGIVING.**

Expect changes in your life, your family members' lives, and Mom's life. To be effective, you must view change as a challenge, not a crisis. Change is normal and motivates many facets of our lives. Change can stimulate and invigorate, and it can lead you to perform in ways not previously considered.

> **If you do not take care of you, how can you expect to provide for Dad's care?**

Get a Handle on Your Emotions

Be prepared. Giving care creates a whole range of emotions, from sadness to anger, from boredom to exhaustion, to joy and pride. Negative feelings (anger, frustration, resentment, etc.) may represent guilt. Doing your best creates nothing to apologize for or feel guilty about, even though sometimes your best is not enough for you or others. Remember it is human to feel anger or resentment as a family caregiver.

Stop Being So Hard on Yourself

If you lose your temper and shout at Grandpa or your little girl who is only trying to help, apologize and move on. If you do that more and more often, however, acknowledge that your "bad temper" is a sign of stress and ask for help. Your biggest mistake would be to falsely assure everyone (including yourself) that you can manage everything on your own. Saying you do not need help or do not want to bother anyone is a normal response in family caregiving, but it is not realistic; eventually *you* will wind up needing a family caregiver if you do not accept support that is offered.

> **Your biggest mistake would be to falsely assure everyone (including yourself) that you can manage everything on your own.**

This *Manual* represents knowledge and experience in nonclinical family caregiving drawn from the experiences of many hundreds of family caregivers and dozens of professionals. Underlying that is the recognition that family caregiving is one of the toughest and most thankless jobs you can undertake. It is also an absolutely necessary job if we are all to receive the care we may one day need. It is also an acknowledgment that there are steps you can take that will not only make you a better caregiver but also will make you a more stable, less stressed, happier person as a family caregiver. You can LEARN better ways to plan for and provide care.

Providing care for others who cannot provide care for themselves places enormous strain on other relationships and responsibilities. Family caregiving and the family caregiver must be respected. No one trains family members in how to engage in resolving long-term problematic events—events that often defy description. Without recognizing what it means, communities and nations expect family caregivers to be the backbone of long-term care and in the front line for loved ones' acute care for the next twenty-five years and probably for always. There is no such thing as the perfect family caregiver. Any family caregiver projecting a standard of perfection defies accomplishment and is destined for failure. No family caregiver is Mother Teresa and Florence Nightingale, so do not set your personal performance bar at the level of a saint or an international paragon of accomplishment—do not set it so high that you can never succeed.

Don't Fear Seeking Comfort When You Need It

Allow your sister June to give back to you emotionally if she is capable of doing so. Being able to give comfort or being asked for her opinion is a wonderful opportunity to participate in something that she may have missed while everyone protected her health and feelings. Sometimes the best gift you can give people made vulnerable by illness or age is the opportunity to have someone need them for a change.

Learn to Laugh at Yourself and with Others

One of your best resources for overcoming negative feelings and guilt is humor. Caregiving is serious business, but you need to step away and enjoy your life if you are going to be effective. Even serious situations have their funny moments. A friend told me that literally moments after her mother died in her arms, a cousin dropped in unannounced who had not visited throughout her mother's illness. When told Mom had just passed, the cousin said, "Well, if I had known she was going to die, I wouldn't have come." What was this cousin thinking? What she said could be viewed as horrible, unfeeling, and disrespectful. My friend, however, who long before had learned to laugh at the absurdity of life, maintained her composure until her cousin walked back down the hall and then laughed until she cried. Her attitude? "Ye gods. Only in our family!"

Seek Peer Support

The importance of attending an appropriate family caregiver support group cannot be overstated. Regularly attending a family caregiver support group offers you (and every family caregiver) the opportunity to

1. find understanding and shared experiences;
2. find out that other people have similar feelings;
3. recognize that you are not the only family caregiver in the world;
4. know that you are not the only one who feels as you do.

Participating in a support group can make the challenge of family caregiving not only tolerable, but also it can lead you to recognize that what you are doing can be personally rewarding.

Do Not Let Stress Win

Can you recognize signs of too much stress? Are you talking louder and faster than normal? Facial expressions, poor posture, lack of emotional control, sleeping disorders, stomach upsets, and headaches are overall signs of stress.

Feeling Stressed? STOP!

Turning off stress is not as easy as saying "Stop!", but there are things you can do that will help you reduce the stress you feel. Take a moment to step away. Look at the situation from all angles. Ask yourself if you truly have any control over the situation and whether there is anything you can you do to change it. If you cannot make a change, do not let stress win. Do not beat yourself up over the uncontrollable. Once you understand the sources of stress, you can take steps toward releasing it. Remember, if you have the Plan in place, you have thought through a number of options that can make things better or at least more workable. Also, if you participate in a family caregiver support group, your fellow caregivers can help you by discussing the stressful situations they faced and how they survived.

Consider these possibilities:

- If stress comes from having to perform an unpleasant task, the best choice may be to **just do it**—the sooner the better—before the stress of the situation becomes greater. Don't put it off. Do it today! Do it now!

- When things pile up, break them into **manageable tasks**. Tackle one task at a time, finish it, and then move on to the next item on the list.

- **Get organized.** Keep the Plan handy so you can refer to it easily to refresh your memory about options. Use lists, calendars, and organizers to track multiple responsibilities. Check your lists often and revise them. Prioritize, putting the "must do" items first, the "do as soon as possible" next, and the "nice to do" items last. Is there anything that can wait or not be done at all? Cross it off.

- **Handle paper only once**. When going through the mail, take the required action immediately—file it, write a check, send a response, or toss it.

- **Learn to delegate**. You cannot do it all.

- **Be open to options.** Get help in the house, have a friend share your load, find a volunteer to stay with the children, or use adult day care or respite.

- **Draw the line.** Even if Uncle Harry objects to having paid help or other family members in the house doing chores, get them in there anyway. Make it clear to Uncle Harry that not having help is not an option. You may have to live with pouting, anger, and attempts to make you feel guilty, but Uncle Harry cannot make you feel guilty or experience negative emotions if you expect his attempts to make that happen and decide not to let his efforts affect you.

- **Relax and take regular breaks**. Stretch after sitting; close your eyes and breathe deeply. Take time to do what you love to do. You have a life—live it!

- **Seeking assistance and support early** increases your family caregiving capability without adversely impacting your life. **Do not wait for a crisis to occur!** Speak up if you feel overwhelmed or unsure how to proceed.

Rate Your Caregiver Stress

Section 1: *First, rate how you perceive the following:*

On a scale of 1 to 10 with 1 being "not stressful" and 10 being "extremely stressful," rate your caregiving situation.	
On a scale of 1 to 10 with 1 being "very healthy" and 10 being "very ill," rate your current health **compared** to last year at this time.	
Total the two ratings here:	

Section 2: *Using the statements below, indicate if you agree or disagree. Be honest! No one else will know.*

	Agree	Disagree
I have trouble keeping my mind on what I am doing.		
I have difficulty making decisions.		
I sometimes feel useless and unneeded.		
My family members feel neglected by me and as if they have no privacy.		
I am upset that my relative/spouse/child/friend has changed so much from his or her former self.		
I am sometimes edgy or irritable.		
My appetite is poor, or I am eating too much.		
I sometimes cry for no apparent reason.		
I have back pain.		
I am dissatisfied with my family's support for me.		
I cannot plan anything; some caregiving problem always interrupts.		

	Agree	Disagree
I feel I can't leave my relative/spouse/child/friend alone for even a short time, as I trust no one to take my place.		
I feel completely overwhelmed.		
Arguments are always going on.		
I feel lonely.		
I have lost my privacy and/or personal time.		
Caregiving activities disturb my sleep.		
My sleep time, even undisturbed, is less than 6 hours.		
I am emotionally distressed by my relative/spouse/child/friend physical problems (e.g. refusal to eat, bathe, incontinence, and untrue accusations).		
I feel strain between work and family responsibilities.		
Money is tight, and there always something else to pay for.		
I made changes at work and I feel my job is in peril.		
I always feel ill.		
The living situation is inconvenient or a barrier to care.		
I don't exercise enough or at all.		
I don't take time for me.		
I feel trapped.		
Count up answers in each column and enter in the boxes on the right.		

How to Interpret Your Scores

Everyone, even noncaregivers, experiences stress.

- **Section 1**, if you rated your caregiving stress at 3 or below, but your health "score" is edging toward 10, discuss your circumstances with a physician. Caregiver stress can kill. Like high blood pressure, it is a silent enemy.

- **Section 2**, the higher the AGREE column score, the greater degree of your stress. Any score below 5 in the AGREE column means you need to look at stress reduction, before it gets worse.

  - If your score is creeping into the teens, take immediate steps to reduce stress.

  - The higher the number in the DISAGREE column, the more likely you have resources to help reduce stress, but you do have stress.

- Stress makes you sick—heart disease, high blood pressure, and other conditions that worsen with stress.

Plan for Stress Reduction

If you acknowledge your stress, you can take steps to reduce and control it. Even if you believe you are experiencing little or no stress now and have never experienced it in the past, as a family caregiver you can anticipate greater stress at various times in the process. Take steps to reduce or prevent stress before it becomes a problem.

Taking care of yourself is a conscious choice.

Do not be like family caregivers who believe they can't take time for themselves. After all, like every family caregiver, they have families to support, work to do, personal needs, and care to provide. Yet, they choose to sacrifice themselves, and because of that they may put themselves, their families, meeting their family caregiving responsibilities, and their loved ones at risk.

Taking care of yourself is a conscious choice. To succeed in family caregiving and also live a positive and healthy life, you need to make that choice. Recognizing the need to take care of you, goes a long way in reducing stress.

So, Be Different

Here are a few proven, stress-reduction suggestions:

- **Use meditation techniques**, such as deep breathing, guided imagery, meditation tapes, massage therapy, and aroma therapy.
- **Exercise daily.** Exercise helps you sleep better and maintain energy levels. Set aside specific times to walk, bike, or swim. Choose activities you enjoy, but be consistent. Even twenty minutes a day can make a real difference.
- **Rest your body and spirit.** Pamper yourself. Nap in the afternoon. Sleep as long as you can each night. Take a hot bath.
- **Do not stifle your creativity.** Learn new things. Continue with hobbies or take up new ones. Enroll in an adult education class. Learning and creativity enriches, energizes, and renews your life.

- **Seek positive people.** Self-help experts call out, "You cannot expect to live a positive life if you hang out with negative people." And they are correct. Negativity breeds negativity. Seek out positive people and share positive experiences.

- **Join a caregiver support group that emphasizes positive solutions.** Find one that understands nonclinical family caregiving. Avoid pity parties that have confirmed beliefs that everything is hopeless, unending, and impossible to endure.

- **Reinforce positive thoughts by using positive affirmations.** Signs saying "I am worthy" and "I deserve good things in life" should be tacked to your mirror or refrigerator. Positive affirmations help combat mild depression and feelings of helplessness.

- **Get organized.** Keep task lists and appointment calendars, and mark deadlines. Try integrating personal and family caregiving business. Banish paper piles (do not keep what you do not need; get a scanner and keep a digital file instead of paper files). Did you get a bill this morning? Act on it. File it. Throw that useless piece of paper away. Keep your living and work space clean. Getting organized helps clear your head, and staying organized keeps it clear. Being organized increases effectiveness and reduces stress.

- **Journal.** Take five or ten minutes at the end of the day to write down events that occurred and feelings you have experienced. Even when you have had a tough day, expressing things in writing can be a positive experience, allowing the release of negative feelings. Reviewing older journals may demonstrate to you that your can-do attitude and efforts are having a positive effect.

- **Do not ignore your health.** Have an annual checkup. Be honest about how you are feeling. Do not blame all aches, pains, and discomforts on family caregiving. If you are not feeling well, remember that everyone has health issues independent of family caregiver stress. Follow your healthcare professional's advice.

- **Eat a balanced, healthy diet.** Include plenty of fruits, fluids, vegetables, and lean proteins. If you do not have a good diet now, remember that following a good diet is a lifestyle change, not just deciding to take in fewer calories. You may wish to consult a nutritionist to help you plan. Limit, or, if you can, eliminate the use of alcohol, tranquilizers, sleeping pills, cigarettes, and recreational drugs.

10.

Understand Continuum of Care

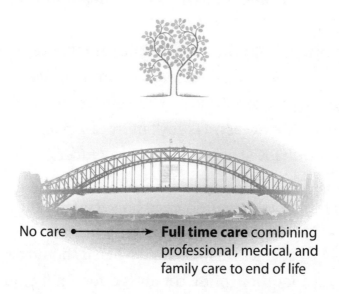

No care ●————→ **Full time care** combining professional, medical, and family care to end of life

The Plan's primary goal is to enable you to prepare and be ready for evolving stages of need along what is called the "continuum of care." Continuum of care is defined as the progression of care provided from wellness through treatment to the end of the need for care—from day one when a health issue presents itself through the last day care is needed. Sometimes, the last day is complete recovery. Sometimes, the last day ends in death.

Once you have prepared your Plan, you will have a clear understanding of where your child, spouse, parent, sibling, or friend is along the continuum and what needs have to be met at whatever stage you are entering into the caregiving process.

As time goes on and things change along the continuum, you will update information and revise and enhance the Plan to address those changes.

Imagine the continuum of care as a bridge over a great river. "No care" is on the left side of the bridge. As the first stage of care begins—and that may constitute nothing more than helping with household chores or keeping a checkbook—you begin to cross the bridge. As you move across, you pass through stages of severity, intensity, and frequency of changing needs. Some things improve, and some worsen. You adapt to the changes. Eventually, you may move all the way across the bridge to a stage of full-time care that combines professional, medical, and family care, and that stage may last until the death of your loved one.

Effective family caregiving begins with seven common necessities.

Regardless of where your loved one is on the bridge, effective family caregiving begins with **seven common necessities** any family caregiver must be able to fulfill:

1. **Communicate** with loved ones and family members.
2. **Interact** with professionals caring for your loved one.
3. **Understand** the clinical condition and how it affects the nature of, demand for, and time required to provide care needs.
4. **Determine** who provides what care and when it should be provided.
5. **Assess** the care location most conducive for safety, quality of life, and convenience.
6. **Calculate** financial resources to pay for care.
7. **Set aside** personal feelings to make practical problem-solving possible. No one makes good practical decisions when emotionally involved. Seek opinions from others not directly involved.

There is an eighth necessity:

8. **Recognize** your own health status and how it affects your capability to care for both yourself and your loved one, and have a clear understanding of what the health status of your loved one is—that is, where he or she is along the continuum.

As ordinary people, we have general ideas about how certain disorders and diseases affect health status. The model below presents one way of looking at health status and provides examples of diseases and conditions that correlate with each status. It is a guide you can adopt, adapt, or ignore.

Effective family caregiving requires a reasonable understanding of the level of care required. You have to be objective to plan effectively if you are a new family caregiver.

MODEL FOR DEFINING HEALTH STATUS

- **Definition 1: Chronic or debilitating condition** requiring ongoing medical care and caregiving that, over time, increasingly limits the ability to act independently.

    Example Conditions: Anemia, thyroid conditions, some hormonal disorders, some forms of heart disease, and controlled diabetes.

- **Definition 2:** Maintaining health **requires self-care** to maintain well-being.

    Example Conditions: Exercise, diet, good sleeping habits, time away, support network, hobbies, spirituality, and preventive care.

- **Definition 3:** Short-term illness or accident with **a positive outcome**.

    Example Conditions: Colds, infections, minor injury, and accidents.

- **Definition 4:** Short-term event leading **to impairment or even death**.

    Example Conditions: Significant illness or accident that requires major medical intervention.

- **Definition 5:** Chronic illness/disorder with **relatively stable caregiving demand**.

    Example Conditions: Intellectual disability, major allergies, conditions controlled and stabilized for long periods of time, and controlled diabetes.

- **Definition 6:** Chronic and **disabling**.

    Example Conditions: MS, lupus, MG, rheumatoid arthritis, dysautonomia, some heart conditions, and dementia-related diseases.

- **Definition 7:** Chronic, disabling, and **terminal over time**.

    Example Conditions: Cancer, AIDS, and advanced heart disease.

How Much Care Is Needed?

There is a difference between care that is needed and care that is wanted by the person being cared for or a family member who feels compelled to provide more care out of a sense of obligation. There are people who need more care than they want to accept and people who want more care than they actually need. There are family members who do not understand how impaired a loved one may be (in spite of any explanation) or want to overly conserve resources. There are family members who are convinced that extra care will delay the inevitable or compensate for their paying too little attention in the past. However, a sound family caregiving Plan is dedicated to planning for needed care and ensuring that it is provided. As a family caregiver, you must always balance what is needed against what is wanted.

Addressing resistance to care has already been discussed a number of times in the *Manual*, but there is a special challenge when a loved one wants more care than he or she needs and, sometimes, more care than can be provided due to setting and limited resources. Receiving special attention can help people overcome their fears, make them feel less isolated, and give them a sense of being loved and belonging. Demanding and having people provide care that is not needed may lend a sense of control and satisfaction, a feeling of still being the boss. In making a decision about whether to provide more care than is needed, consider what is best for your loved one in the long run. When a person is capable of taking care of his/her own needs, it is important that he/she continues to do so in order to maintain independence and capability for as long as possible. There is a certain truth in the concept of "use it or lose it."

Once you understand what is needed and what it will take to make sure needed care is provided, you can then decide whether to provide additional care based on available resources.

Determining Need

To plan, think in terms of the ability of your loved one to perform tasks now and in the future; factor in what is likely to happen due to increasing physical, emotional, and practical challenges. The following ten-point scale can help you decide, first, where your loved one's capability is now and, second, what is likely to change over time.

When looking at the scale, consider what is normal for the age group your loved one falls into (e.g., four years old, ten years old, fifteen years old, twenty years old, eighty years old). What is "normal" for one age group is vastly different for what is "normal" for another. Physical, mental, emotional, social, and other needs differ.

Also, consider the nature of what your loved one is experiencing. Steps to be taken and care needs differ depending on what the issues are. When a chronic and progressive disorder is involved, care needs are likely to increase at the same pace as the effects of the disorder. When a sudden and debilitating physical change occurs, for instance, as the result of sudden-onset illness, an accident, or a war injury, one day things can be normal and the next day full-time care and huge demands on resources may be needed. In family caregiving, although you can plan ahead, timing is everything!

> **Remember:** The seven necessities listed earlier in this chapter must always be addressed regardless of age or illness. The greater the degree of required action, the greater the need is to act quickly and intelligently. Developing the Plan when there is no crisis is far better than having to make rapid decisions under stress.

LEVELS OF NEED

Level 1

There is no evidence of disease or need for care. Your loved one is able to work, play, and interact without any concern. You are just planning ahead.

Level 2

Your loved one is performing normal activities, but there are some minor signs of change, a few complaints, and a few signs or symptoms of illness. Plans need to include evaluating what is going on and implementing a preventative strategy, as well as considering what may happen later.

Level 3

The signs and symptoms of a change in physical and/or mental well-being are obvious. Your loved one is still maintaining his or her normal lifestyle, but it is clear that he or she is using more effort to play, work, and stay engaged socially. Plans need to include medical evaluation and possibly preventive care or intervention and looking at resources to ensure that anticipated needs can definitely be met in the future.

Level 4

Your loved one is unable to carry on normal activities but can still provide self-care. Medical care is ongoing and more attention must be paid to maintaining self-care in the home.

Level 5

Your loved one requires occasional assistance but is able to care for most personal needs. The assistance of a family caregiver or paid caregiver is being used. More concrete planning should be done for future needs.

Level 6

Your loved one requires considerable assistance and frequent medical care. More hours are spent in providing needed assistance. You need to review and modify the Plan more frequently and monitor the use of resources on a regular basis. Parts of the Plan are being activated more frequently.

Level 7

Your loved one is disabled and requires special care and assistance. The family is now engaged in very active family caregiving, and the home is now the site of full-fledged caregiving. The disease or disability is likely progressing rapidly, and changes in need occur frequently. Planning needs to anticipate full-time, complex care in the home. It may be necessary to provide institutional care because needs cannot be met in the home.

Level 8

Your loved one is severely disabled. Hospitalization at least for a period of time or institutional care is needed. Care cannot be maintained in the home unless major improvements are made, but even then twenty-four-hour care will be necessary. Planning must address twenty-four-hour care, most likely in an institutional setting, or at least delivered in the home.

Level 9

Your loved one is very sick, and you cannot care for him or her at home without major in-home care assistance, as stated above, or hospice care. Transfer to institutional care may be the best option. Hospital treatment may be needed, but regardless consideration needs to be given to end-of-life issues such as your loved one's preferences regarding taking extreme measure to maintain life.

Level 10

Your loved one is approaching the end of life rapidly. He or she is "shutting down," and death is imminent. His or her preferences for end-of-life care have been implemented. This may include dying at home or in an institutional setting, but your loved one is most likely under hospice care and is definitely being continually monitored medically. The Plan should be reviewed related to funeral plans.

ADDITIONAL CONSIDERATIONS

On the following pages are a few additional points for consideration related to planning for needs. If you have questions about what should be done in detail, review the *Manual* chapters to refresh your memory. If you already have your Plan prepared, review the Plan. Talk to family members. You can also discuss matters with your professional caregiving advisor.

If Your Loved One's Need Is Level 1 through 3

Even if your loved one has some signs and symptoms of disease, he or she is able to carry out normal activities.

- Your Plan should be prepared by now; if not, prepare it. Review and revise, as needed, any existing Plan and supporting documentation to be sure everything that is needed is in place and planned actions are up to date.
- Make sure that everyone who as agreed to support caregiving is ready.

If Your Loved One's Need Is Level 4 through 6

At this rating level, your loved one requires assistance. At the highest level (6), he or she needs considerable assistance and frequent medical care.

- Review the Plan and supporting documentation to be sure everything that is needed is in place and planned actions are up to date.
- If Advanced Directives and Durable Powers of Attorney have not been created, now it is absolutely essential that the documents are prepared as quickly as possible.
- Schedule a family update and prepare them for implementing their part of the Plan.

If Your Loved One's Need Is Level 7

Your loved one is now in the range of requiring serious family caregiving.

- Include all the steps outlined previously.
- Spend time discussing care needs (when, where, what) with the medical team.
- Put planned services that are needed into place.

If Your Loved One's Need Is Level 8 through 10

Likely you are deep into family caregiving and may be going in and out of crisis. Obviously, everything said about levels 4 through 7 applies, as well as the following:

- It may be time to place full-time care in the home; if so, begin the hiring process. If facility-based care is more appropriate, implement the part of the Plan that covers placement.
- Are pre-need funeral arrangements made and in order?
- Has hospice care and other end-of-life considerations been discussed? Is it now necessary to bring in hospice?

- Work with the medical team to ensure you are updated and when the time for discharge comes, get a copy of the discharge Plan of Care. Ask for as much lead time as possible prior to discharge from a hospital or facility.

Note: If your loved one is not yet ready, or needed care is not available, you have an absolute right to dispute a discharge, ask for a review, and appeal from the review. Make sure you understand the process. As a family caregiver, if the burden that would be placed on you by the formal healthcare system is not practical and/or sustainable, then providing care at home is out of the question. The role of family caregiver pushes you to your limits, but expecting you to do the impossible is not a reasonable expectation.

Beyond Level 10

What happens after your loved one no longer needs your care? There probably should be an eleventh level of need on the scale—one that relates to you and your family members who survive the death of a loved one.

Family caregiving and planning do not actually end with death and a funeral. Planning for needs should include issues such as grief counseling for survivors, handling estate issues, and revising everyone's personal care Plan to reflect such a major change as the loss of a loved one.

Many family caregivers have been in the role for an extended period of time. The routine and responsibility can become "addictive"; therefore, withdrawing from caregiving is neither easy nor quick.

When you are suddenly no longer a family caregiver, you have also lost your "job" and identity, and those losses compound and exacerbate the grief and sense of loss from the physical loss of your loved one.

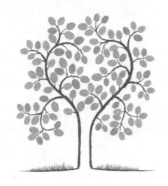

11.

Write Your Plan/Make It Work

*"In the world of family caregiving, if
something can go wrong, it will!"*
X—The world's first family caregiver

When talking with your advisor or reading the *Manual*, you
have been told how important it is to prepare a plan, and that a
written plan can be prepared and revised as needs arise. You have
been told that having a written plan can make it much easier to
decide what steps to take next. And, you have spent a good deal of
time considering the real needs of your loved one and gathering
information about resources. You have a lot of information at
your fingertips. But just how do you prepare a written plan that
organizes that information and makes it really useful?

Putting ideas down on paper is never easy—even professional writers can have
problems expressing themselves. For you, as a family caregiver, the goal should be
to put your ideas down in an orderly way so that YOU (and perhaps others in your
family) can use what you write as a tool, not just for planning, but also for making
your plan work.

The following ideas will help you make decisions about how to write your plan.

What Should Your Plan Look Like?

Language and Writing Skills

Do not worry about whether you are a good writer or not. You can use complete sentences like "Contact Dr. Brown and request more information on the level of pain medication to administer," or write in phrases like "call dr re pain med dosage." The most important thing is that you and the other people who use the Plan can understand what has to be done. Concern yourself with being clear about what you want to happen in the days to come.

You are not being graded on your writing ability. You may have a Master's degree in English or English may be your second language. You may never have gotten past fifth grade writing. Write in the style you are most comfortable with. If you can't write then try and work with a trusted person who can join you in creating the Plan and may be better at putting the words on paper. No one is going to come along and give you a "grade." You may have terrible handwriting—no one cares as long as you can read it. Afterward, you can always get help in putting it all together. This is important in case others need to use your Plan and information if you are not available. If everyone in the family speaks a language other than English and some do not speak English at all, and you are the caregiver who is writing the Plan, having a version in the other language will help everyone else understand what to do. If someone who has to use the Plan is visually impaired or has limited or no ability to read or write, be prepared to explain the Plan in detail so that person understands what must be done and when. You could also make an audio recording that could be sent to one or more people to listen to, and they could then ask you questions.

There is a sample plan at the end of this chapter. It is written in what is called "narrative form"; it contains complete sentences and regular paragraphs. It was typed on a computer so it could be revised and printed repeatedly. You might be more comfortable writing out a plan by hand and making photocopies for people who need them. You may want to create bulleted lists. For example, you could list your personal life goals like this:

My Goals

- *Have at least one evening during the week and one day on the weekend to do what I want to do (go to movie, go fishing).*
- *Get the dental work I need done within six months.*
- *No more meals over the sink; sit down at the table to eat.*

What Order Should You Put the Information?

The simple answer is to put the information in an order that works for you. However, if you have gathered information in the order it is listed in Chapter Six or if you used the Family Caregiver Questionnaire, it might be easier to put the information in the order of the questions you answered.

If you look at the sample at the end of this chapter, you will notice that the writer begins by providing information about herself as a caregiver—family background and health information, and so on. This person used a version of the Family Caregiving Questionnaire to gather her information and then to guide her as she thought about what she needed to do.

How Much Information Should You Include?

The woman who wrote the sample was selective about what she included in the actual Plan. Much of the information she collected (e.g., details about insurance plans and available resources) helped her identify problems she needed to address, but she did not include all the details. The Family Caregiver Questionnaire is like an encyclopedia—it is a collection point for a lot of information that can be useful but doesn't have to be repeated.

Say what is necessary to make the plan clear, for example, "The health policy Dad has limits out-of-pocket expenses to $2,000 a year, but there is a cap on lifetime expenses for day care of $100,000. Report expenses monthly." You do not have to say, "Mail expenses to [company name and mailing address]," but you can always look the information up on the Family Caregiver Questionnaire or refer to the actual policy.

Keeping these important points in mind as you work on your Plan will make your task easier. Before you begin to write, review what you learned in each of the chapters and the information you gathered using the Family Caregiver Questionnaire:

- **Chapter 1** helped you define yourself as a family caregiver.

- **Chapter 2** provided case examples of individuals who were faced with a need to do care planning. The observations about each case should have helped you begin to think about questions you needed to answer in your own Plan.

- **Chapter 3** emphasized the importance of having a positive attitude about being a family caregiver and about the ways guilt and resentment can affect your attitude. It also discussed ways to help maintain that positive attitude, including attending a family caregiver support group.

- **Chapter 4** discussed keys to successful planning.

- **Chapter 5** explained the benefits of documenting lifestyle, medical, and financial information and how that information was necessary to understand how to meet family caregiving needs.

- **Chapter 6** provided a very detailed list of items you could include in documentation, including income and expenses items. As you gather information, remember to do the following:

  - **Take your time**. Assembling data and information may take awhile and involve making requests of others (e.g., doctor, Medicare, VA, family members, lawyer, financial planner).

  - **Ask the family and neighbors, as well as your loved one, for missing information.** It is essential to the Plan to have an accurate assessment of what the family history is. You don't need extensive details, but it is important to know what illnesses, if any, your loved one's parents, grandparents, aunts, uncles suffered from. Did your family have any psychological issues? Did anyone in the family have children who died at an early age (From what? How old?)? If your loved served in the military or in a stressful work situation (coal miner, security guard, police officer, etc.) that could contribute to a psychological issue today or in the near future.

  - **Be accurate in your assessment of family attitudes and resources.** Determine whether "old issues" may prevent your family members from being accurate or even participating in fact gathering. There may be deep-seated and long-standing resentments that you are not aware of but may contribute to the effectiveness of your Plan or have play a part in your loved one's care, attitude, and setting for care.

- **Gather supporting documents** (e.g., healthcare directives) so you have complete records and the paperwork you need to make things happen.

- **Strive for accuracy, but remember there is no such thing as perfection.** Your efforts may leave gaps that become obvious as you try and put the information together in a meaningful way. Don't worry; planning is an ongoing effort, and over time gaps may disappear. If the information is not available, however, it simply isn't available. You will adapt.

▪ **Chapter 7** covered getting organized, family meetings, and things you need to consider when deciding about care needs.

▪ **Chapter 8** reviewed issues that involve practical problem solving, such as health options, questions to ask the doctor, housing (including making decisions about renovation and safety issues), and how to hire in-home support.

▪ **Chapter 9** talked about YOU and how you can take better care of yourself.

▪ **Chapter 10** defined the concept of the continuum of care and how the information you are gathering defines your loved one's position on the continuum and the plans you put into place to address the needs of today and tomorrow.

▪ **The Family Caregiver Questionnaire**: Look at each section. Do you have all the information you need? If not, do you have enough to begin writing about the part of the Plan that requires this information? If information is missing, you can make another attempt to collect it before writing your Plan, but don't delay too long even if you are missing some of the details— you can always add information later. You may also decide that you have all the information about a topic you can reasonably get and should not delay writing the Plan. You can also use the structure of the Family Caregiver Questionnaire as an outline for your Plan.

Part 1: The Caregiver's List: This section includes current information about **you** (e.g., contact information, tasks you perform as a caregiver). The section on your goals as a caregiver is especially important. The Plan will work best when your goals AND the needs of your loved one are met at the same time.

Part II: The Person Needing Care Now or in the Future: This section provides great detail on your loved one's way of living and care needs—personal data (including a recent photo), living situation, pets, health issues, and medical issues—all the things that make the person you are caring for the person he or she is and the things that help determine how you interact with him or her as a family caregiver. Do not overlook the importance of including issues that may arise related to family medical history. If this person is also a family caregiver, be sure to include information on his or her caregiving responsibilities and how they will be handled if your loved one is unable to perform those tasks.

Financial and Legal Information: This section includes lists of documents; locations of papers, passwords, and account numbers; lists of professionals used by your loved one; bills and how they are paid; bank addresses; and so on. Much of this information is useful in just managing daily living, but information about insurance coverage, monthly income, monthly expenses, and so on is vital to evaluating the resources you have available. When preparing your plan, you don't have to repeat every detail of this information. However, you need to consider it in relation to how if effects the choices you make. Be sure to keep original documents in a safe place that is easily accessible in a crisis. The section on monthly income and expenses is critical to your Plan.

Important points to remember:

1. **Every family caregiving Plan is different. Your Plan will be unique to your situation.** Your plan should discuss what your personal family caregiving experience is like, what the people are like, whose attitudes and opinions need to be considered, and other factors that you (and your advisor) believe to be important. Remember—*this is only an example.*

2. **Be prepared for change.** When everything in the *Manual* is taken into account, the foundation for effective planning and understanding options is clearer. However, nothing could be truer than the adage "The best laid plans . . . often go awry." If you have more than one option to solve a problem, include all the options (so you don't forget), and if one option doesn't work, you won't have to work hard to look at other options—they will be right there in the Plan.

Expect things to happen, good and bad, that you do not expect to happen right now. You may have to change course in mid-stream or face a problem you have never seen before. Regardless, the information you have gathered in the process of using the *Manual* and preparing your Plan will be helpful to you as you face next challenges. Update your Plan to reflect changes that occur and be prepared to change your mind about what you should do. One of the keys to effective family caregiving is adaptability. If you are prepared for change, change is not as stressful and you will make better decisions.

3. **If your Plan cannot be implemented due to financial constraints, it is not a usable Plan.** Simply put, if all you have is a dime to spend, do not create a Plan that requires you to spend a dollar.

4. **Be patient if you are waiting for information, but start your plan as soon as you have basic information in hand.** If you are in a crisis situation, you may have to work really hard to get the information you need immediately. However, in general, keep in mind that assembling the information you need may take some time, and people who have the information you need may take a long time to respond. For example, if you want a veteran's record, weeks may pass before the VA responds to your request.

> **If all you have is a dime to spend, do not create a Plan that requires you to spend a dollar.**

5. **You don't have to sit down and write the whole Plan at once.** Even an experienced caregiving advisor typically writes a Plan in sections. Take some of the easy stuff first. For example, you might describe your family history and talk about close relatives. You could skip to a bit of medical information and talk about primary physicians and what they treat. You could list your most important personal goals as a caregiver. Remember, your loved one's needs did not develop in a day or a week or even a year. There is no reason to think you have to prepare the final Plan in an hour. However, do keep in mind that you need that first version, and sooner is better than later. You may need a Plan for handling a crisis, sooner than you think.

6. **Be sensitive to how your loved one and other family members may feel about the information you have gathered.** In the process of researching family information and medical histories, you may have discovered very personal information about your family and your loved one. You will know a lot about financial issues that many others do not know and have information on health issues that people may consider very private. For

example, you may find out that an uncle who is a pillar of the community has a criminal record that was long buried or belonged to organizations that at one time may have seemed appropriate but in today's society would be objectionable.

As you gather information you need to decide how information relates to what the Plan is about—how best to provide for the essential care of a loved one in the future—and whether it needs to be or should be shared with people who may use the Plan and help with care over time. Be discrete and careful about what you say and how you say it. When in doubt, leave it out, but keep it in your raw data file in case the information should be needed later to explain something or becomes important in providing care or treatment, facility placement, and other circumstances.

7. **After you prepare the first Plan, have someone else look at it.** This person could be someone who shares care responsibilities or a trusted neighbor or a professional advisor. Ask your reviewer to look for things that are confusing or seem to be incomplete. Ask the person whether he or she could take the plan and follow it if necessary. In other words, have them be your "editor." Once you get feedback, go back and fix things before you share the plan with anyone else.

8. **Finally, remember *why* you are doing what you are doing.** The object of all the work you are doing and have done to create the Plan is for you to be able to understand the options that are available in caring for your loved one and make the best decisions you can. Sometimes, and maybe always, the options will be lousy and not what you would have wanted. However, in developing the Plan you will learn what you have to work with, and that will help you feel confident you are making the best decisions you can make at the time you have to decide. With this knowledge this comes the peace of mind you did the best you could with what you had to work with and that no one could have done better. **Creating the Plan is critical.**

Even if the unexpected arises, do not abandon the Plan.
Just be prepared for the unplanned.
Remember, you are not alone; millions face family caregiving.
However, few have planned ahead—you have.
Good luck and good planning!

Sample Narrative and Plan

This plan was written by a real unpaid family caregiver. The names of the caregiver, her husband, and her family caregiving advisor and the actual location in which the caregiver lives have been changed. No other changes have been made.

Date Written: January 19, 2014

This plan is about my Mother, Alice Baker Simms.

My name is Mary Ellen Tucker. I take care of my mother and my husband. Ms. Cedra Plank, my family caregiver professional, is helping me prepare this plan. She is also advising me in how to be a better family caregiver for my mother and my husband. The information I am using comes from the worksheets that Cedra gave me a few weeks ago. I finished them last night. In assembling the information and in writing small pieces of this plan before Cedra and I started working together today, I already understand more about what I am facing with my mom. I expect that Cedra and I will put together what Cedra calls a "nonclinical" Family Caregiving Plan for Mother. Because of the preparation I have done for Mother's plan, I see a real value in doing this kind of thing and after we finish this plan for Mother, Cedra and I will work on a plan for my husband. Planning this way will help me help both of them without becoming an emotional and physical burn out from doing way too much family caregiving.

I took the Family Caregiver tests that Cedra gave me, and it showed that I am not too stressed right now and I guess that is true. The other part of the test said that I am a good problem solver, like I always thought. As I got ready to do this plan, I also realized that solving problems for my husband and about my house is a lot different than solving problems that come up where Mother is concerned. After thinking about it, I realized that she is far less cooperative than I thought she was going to be when this all started. She has a very negative attitude and is "stubborn as a mule," and my assumption that under the circumstances she would listen to me or her doctor, Dr. Thorne, seems to be wrong.

I also found out something else through all this. When Cedra gave me the Manual, I finally found out what a family caregiver really is and that my role is far more than daughter and wife where my Mom and my husband are concerned. According to the definitions, I am a local, alpha primary family caregiver. That is a mouthful, but I think it means I am the local family caregiver (not long distance) the primary person responsible for looking after both of them and I am also the lead decision maker (alpha) as my brother cannot assume that role.

Here is a little bit of information about me and my husband. I am 62. I have been married to C.W.—his full name is Cletus Williams Tucker—for 40 years. He and I are the same age. We live in Templar, Illinois, and both of us grew up near here in Garrison.

We have two grown children, Nancy who's 34 and Sally Mae who's 38. Nancy married Jack Calhoun when she was 20 and has two children. She and Jack are Lutheran missionaries in Senegal, Africa. They have another 3 years on their assignment there. Sally lives in Australia where she works for a software company. She's never been married.

So, I don't see either of the girls much more than once every three or four years and don't expect to see my grandkids until the oldest one is 15 or 16. I miss them all a lot, especially because I can't watch Nancy's girl and boy grow up. I once thought about visiting in Africa, but that is not going to happen now. My health is fair, but I have a few concerns. I had a radical mastectomy 10 years ago and have a familial tremor. And, I do get tired a lot more easily than I used to do. The internet helps me stay in touch with them.

My husband worked for the Phelps Corrugated Box Company up in Banner until an accident three years ago. A lift full of heavy cardboard toppled over onto his hips and legs. He's on permanent disability now and can't work. He has had four operations on his hips and legs and goes to a pain clinic. He also has to wear a colostomy bag because of the accident. And, he has other problems—he's 40 pounds overweight and has high blood pressure, and I can tell he's depressed. Like I said above, I'm his family caregiver and Mother's.

We live in a two-story house in Templar, and she lives over in Garrison, about eight miles from here. I taught elementary school for 38 years but "retired" 2 ½ years ago so I could help my husband full time. We have rearranged the house so that the dining room is a bedroom for him because he can't climb stairs since the accident. I worry that if he falls I will never be able to lift him. It happened once, and I had to call 911. Fortunately, he wasn't hurt then, but it could happen if he falls again. So much for me and my husband—I need a whole other plan to say everything there is to say about us and, believe me, it will be done!

About Mother. My Mother, Alice, is 82 years old. She's part English (mostly) and part Irish. She was born in Garrison, Illinois, on September 8, 1932. She was born a Baker and was the youngest of the six children her mom and dad—Hilda and Jack Baker—had. Grandpa Jack was an engineer on the Illinois Central Railroad, and Grandma Hilda was a stay at home mom, at least for a while. She told us that when Grandpa died of pleurisy he was only 42. Grandma Hilda had to go to work so she could raise my mother and my aunts and uncles. She worked at a cereal plant in Garrison until she retired at 65. She lived to be 88 and died in 1987, at home, with what we think was Alzheimer's. My mother took care of her the whole time. I don't think she ever got rested up after Grandma Hilda passed.

My mother was also the youngest child in the family. She had three brothers and two sisters who were older. Starting with the oldest after her there was Marie, Jack, Jr., Celia, Fred, and Albert. Jack, Jr., died in a car crash when he was 19, not too long after WWII. Fred died at age 58 of complications from pneumonia and his congestive heart failure. Albert died in 2007 at 77 of a heart attack. Marie died in 2009 at 82; she got some kind of an infection after she had surgery for her broken hip and never left the hospital. Aunt Celia was really sweet, but she had a really hard life because she had what I now understand is a mental condition called bi-polar (we just thought she was "tetched in the head") and then she got Alzheimer's real bad. She died in 2007 in a nursing home in Joliet when she was 78.

My dad, Sam Clayton Simms, was named after his grandfather, but I don't know much about his family, and Mother doesn't remember much. He was orphaned in his teens. My parents met at a USO club during the Korean War and got married in 1952 when Dad got out of the Army. They bought a house in Garrison near Grandma Hilda's place and that was where I was born. My brother Edward was born in the new hospital a year later. He's 61. Like Grandpa Jack, my dad went to work for the Illinois Central after Korea, and he was killed in a derailment in 1977. Mom got a widow's benefit each month but kept her job working as a secretary at the First Bank of Garrison until she retired at 65 and then kept busy working in the Woolworth's until she was 75. She stopped work when they closed the store.

Mother's been going to the Garrison Advent Lutheran Church since she was a kid and was real active at the church until a couple of years ago. The Pastor visits her often, and she has always told him she was going to do "something good" for Advent when she's gone. She still lives alone in the same small home in Garrison that I was born in. She tries to do all the housework but does tell me she lets her neighbors help out some "as a kindness to them." She won't ever say she can't manage by herself. She has two cats that are getting on in years like the rest of us and a mutt dog she named Shem after she found him in the drain pipe that runs under the road in front of her house.

The house is over 75 years old now and needs a lot of work—a new roof, the electric is shot, and it still has a coal bin and coal furnace. It's on a real nice piece of land, about 7 acres I think, over there next to the new expressway interchange. I had one of C.W.'s friends take a look at the house because he is a contractor, and he gave me an estimate of what it would take to repair the place and change out the heating system for an oil burner and get everything else into shape. He said that with the new roof with a new oil furnace and with all of the upgrades needed we were looking at around $65,000.00. I never mentioned this number to Mother; she'd have a stroke on top of everything else that's wrong.

My brother Ed can't help much, but he tries to visit Mom at least once a year. He's a salesman for an adhesive company and travels a lot. He lives in St. Louis with his second wife Selma. His first wife died the first year they were married from a malignant brain tumor. He has two kids, his son Kent from Selma's first marriage and a daughter from their marriage named Eleanor Darla Simms. Selma has MS real bad and is bed bound, and my brother spends most of his time worrying about her care or worrying about how to pay for it. Most of Selma's meds are not covered by my brother's medical insurance from work. He is always fighting with them. The really terrible thing is Eleanor, who is unmarried and has stayed at home since after college to take care of my sister-in-law (now for more than thirteen years because my brother is on the road). Eleanor is only 35 and is showing serious signs of MS as well.

Dr. Thorne has been Mother's primary doctor for over 30 years. She trusts him about everything, even if she won't listen to him. He has already diagnosed her with high blood pressure, arthritis, osteoporosis, and cataracts, and she walks with a limp from a bad car accident years ago. That's her fault because, as stubborn as she is, she didn't follow his orders about rehab when she got hurt and her foot never healed right. The way she walks on that bad foot throws her back off, and she has serious curvature of the spine that's getting worse. She uses a cane and tires real easily but is too proud to use a wheelchair. Dr. Thorne has warned her time and again that she needs surgery for her cataracts and that she's going to slip and fall if she stays in the house by herself. She sees a rheumatologist, Dr. Randall Creighton, and he is treating her arthritis and back problems. I don't know him, but Mom says he's a real good doctor. Dr. Throne and Dr. Creighton have tried to get Mom to see a cardiologist, but she insists that she is happy with her treatment from them. Dr. Thorne has told me that they are both concerned because she basically ignores her high blood pressure. They have prescribed for it but think its bad enough for her to go to a cardiologist so he can treat her heart correctly. Three years ago she had pneumonia and was put in the hospital, and while she was there the hospital sent in a cardiologist to look at her. He thought her heart might be enlarged. It was just like her that even after he told her it could be bad, she just left the hospital and she never went to see him.

Mother is taking 6 different medicines, 4 by prescription and 3 over the counter. Mother has lost some weight recently, and Dr. Thorne noted that she has gone from 122 pounds (her consistent weight for the past five years) to 117 pounds. I have noticed that she just nibbles on her food lately and does not seem to have the same desire for eating that she has always had.

She takes the following medications:

1. High blood pressure – Atenolol
2. Arthritis – Cyclosporine
3. Cataracts – over the counter eye drops
4. Back Injury – Prescription NSAIDS and oxycodone
5. Osteoporosis – Calcium Supplement / OsCal
6. Multivitamins

Mother still enjoys her glass of whiskey before bed. She said it makes the pills go down easier. I asked, "Which pills?"—"the ones for pain" she said, which scares me considering what I have heard about mixing liquor and pills.

When I took her to see Dr. Throne 3 months ago, I told him that I have noticed she's more forgetful. When I take her grocery shopping she gets disoriented in the aisles. This is the same store and same isles she has been shopping at for the last 15 years. He told me to keep a diary on Mom's activities with times of day and circumstances when she has trouble remembering, keeping in mind that the cataracts make it hard for her to see. She has trouble walking, and I am supposed to try to gauge how tired she is and whether she is tiring more quickly. I said I would. Now that I'm keeping this diary, I can see that she is failing a little more than I had realized. Looking at the schedule I keep with her, I have also realized there is no schedule—everything is based on when she wants something done and is very haphazard. It's not the best use of my time and makes it hard for me to get other things done.

She has a Last Will and Testament but keeps it in the safety box at the First National Bank in Garrison. No one has a key except her, and she's never added me or my brother to the list of people who can have access to it. She took me to the bank one day and opened the box. She's got a lot of jewelry left to her by her two sisters and one very old 20-dollar gold coin called a South Panama Pacific dated 1915. She has no idea where Dad got it or when, but she told me that my father had it appraised years ago and it was worth almost $10,000. I recently looked the coin up on the internet and was amazed when I found one I think was like it on sale for $100,000. I haven't told anyone in the family about that, but I asked my mother what she wanted done with the jewelry and the coin and she said it's all in the will. I asked her if I could see it (the will) and she said it was "bad luck" to do that. 3 years ago Mother had a bad bout of pneumonia and was hospitalized in New Slattery at St. Mary's Hospital about 30 miles from home. Dr. Throne was not on staff there and when I tried to get information from the attending doctor, she asked me for my mother's power of attorney and something called a designation of healthcare proxy. I had neither (still don't) and until Dr. Throne called, I could not get much information on her condition. They asked Mother if she had a living will, and she said she had a will. When re-asked if she had a living will she said, "Why do I need a will when I'm still alive?" They asked if she would execute a Do Not Resuscitate order and she said, "I came to the hospital to live and not to die." She is very stubborn. Once I found out from Cedra how important having all these documents can be (the need for a Healthcare Proxy and a Durable Power of Attorney and Advanced Directives) and knowing that she won't listen to me, I asked Dr. Throne to discuss this with her. She told him she would consider it, but there didn't seem to be a rush. She told him that when she was at St. Mary's she did "just fine" without them.

I checked off a lot of chores that I do on the caregiver's checklist Cedra gave me, and the list just seems to grow. I call Mother once or twice a day and go by there almost every day. I take her to her doctor appointments and most of the time I take her to the food store and drug store. Sometimes a neighbor does that but not very often. Her eyes are so bad that I write the checks out for her bills most of the time, but she insists on signing all of them even if I have to show her where every time. I vacuum and dust and do laundry when I can but see that I will have to do more housekeeping, maybe all of it, if she stays in the house. She was forced to give up driving 5 years ago and relies mostly on me and her church friends to get around. There's no town bus out where she lives and no van service in our area for the elderly like some places have. She doesn't get out much, except every once in a while to church but talks a bit on the phone. Ted King has been delivering her mail for 15 years, and getting the mail is the highlight of her day.

She has a handy man, Lester Oakes, and he does basic chores for her and keeps the acreage mowed and does the best he can to keep the house in reasonable condition. Mom won't spend anything to repair the place, so his hands are tied. If things get desperate, I try to scrape together enough to pay for what has to be done. He shovels coal in the furnace for her, but he is getting a little too old to keep doing that.

Mother's finances are all over the place, and I am still trying to track down a few things. She is so secretive about her money, but since I have to help her get her income tax prepared each year (and assemble the papers) I have a basic idea.

She has a bit put away in one form or another. She paid up a life insurance policy for $50,000 while she worked and that could be cashed in for $47,000. That policy is in the safe box with her stock shares. When Aunt Marie died in '04, she left Mom her 1000 shares of stock in Illinois Oil. Back then those shares were worth about a $5,000. She's kept them in the safe box since then. According to the paper, the stock is now worth about $125,000. She has a CD of my father's that she rolls over every 5 years since he died, and it is worth about $110,000. She refuses to touch that money. What really surprised me is that she has a checking account with approximately $37,000 in it. I am not sure where that all came from except that she saved about $15,000 before she retired. As far as I know Mother hasn't put any money away since then. If things get bad for her, I am not sure what we would do. From what I understand, nursing homes cost a lot, assuming we could get her to go to one. There is some real estate—an old cottage she and Dad bought on Stilton Lake about 60 miles away that has a tenant. The tenant made an offer to buy the cottage about 6 weeks ago, but Mother didn't respond yet. The tenant offered $145,000 for the cottage (I know because I had to read her the offer). Mother has no idea what it's worth (it has been in the family since a few years after I was born) and neither do I.

Lester, the handy man, told me recently that when he was cutting the field, some men came up to him and asked who owned the land. They told him they were interested in buying the property, so Lester sent them up to the house to talk to Mom. She told them that what she would do with the property is all in her will. They left a card.

I just found out that she planned out her funeral in detail down to the dress she wants to be buried in and made all of the arrangements with her church and at Ames Funeral Parlor. She has one of those prepaid funerals with them and will be buried next to my dad.

She gets about 4 dividend checks a year from the shares, and last year it added up to about $23,000 that she saved for things like property tax; that went pretty quickly between the tax and the clothes washer she had to buy this year. Mother gets $873 in Social Security after the Medicare is taken out and that old widow's pension from the railroad at $483. She rents out the cottage for about $350. That only comes to $1,700 or so a month, but she gets another $200 deposited from somewhere into her bank account each month. I haven't found out where that comes from yet. She may have other assets, but she never talks about it. So, she manages on about $1,900 a month and so far that works.

At first I thought what she has sounded like a lot, but without selling stock or land, cash to pay bills is actually getting pretty tight, what with the way things are right now, and then there are her medical deductibles. She has fee-for-service Medicare and one of those supplemental policies from AARP that costs $202.50 per month. She has well water (those pipes into the house are always freezing up in the winter), but her other utilities (electric for the lights and some baseboard heat, the cost of coal) run another $300 or so a month. She gets most of her medication from the railroad health plan mail order dispensary but spends about $20 a month on over-the-counter. She spends $1200 per month for food, house supplies, Lester's services, church, and her few charities. Telephone is $35.00 for basic service. That totals about $1,750 a month, leaving her about $150 extra. For the last five years she has saved $100 per month on average so she can buy things for birthdays and Christmas.

Basic Analysis:

1. Mother is 82 and has a family history of cardiac disease and Alzheimer's disease, and she has had cardiac problems for years and is beginning to show signs of dementia (Alzheimer's). Her not getting care from a heart doctor for her heart problems is a real problem and has to be taken care of now.

2. Her other problems—poor eyesight, arthritis, osteoporosis, and orthopedic problems—make her ability to live at home alone a real concern and an issue that must be resolved soon.

3. She has no independent support system short of the handyman and an occasional neighbor. There is no other family member who can pitch in other than me. I am already caring for my husband and cannot devote the time and attention Mother needs to remain at home. I cannot have her move in because our house is already modified to take care of my husband, and there is no more room on the first floor. There isn't enough room in her house for live-in help if we could find it and afford it, and the house is not in good enough condition to have someone live in even if there was room and money for live-in help.

4. There aren't many places around here where Mom could go, but several of Mom's women friends from the church are living at the Lutheran Retirement Home in Kingston (25 miles away). Maybe they would help to persuade her

to consider a move over there. I need to ask the Pastor about the place and see if he would go with me to talk to them.

5. The lack of the legal paperwork is the biggest problem after her health. I think I need to try to get the Pastor to tell her that sharing the will and getting all those powers of attorneys and other things done is the "right thing to do" because not doing it creates problems for me when I try to talk to doctors and work with the bank.

6. I need to contact her attorney to see who should draw up her Durable Powers of Attorney and Living Will and if there is any other paper work, including a lease or contract for the lakeside cabin. I also need to ask him if there are other railroad benefits for widows that we never applied for. If they have a benefit that could supplement the cash she gets, maybe she could go into the Lutheran Home without having to use other money she has until we get the right paperwork done.

7. **Very important:** Get the same paperwork done for me and my husband, but I need someone other than one of our daughters to be that healthcare surrogate because both of them live so far away.

8. Get in touch with Ken Broodmare, C.W.'s real estate agent friend from the Lodge, and see about whether we can sell the house and land and what the value might be since it is so close to the interchange.

9. Get him to give us the name of a real estate agent over around Stilton Lake and see what the value of the lake cottage might really be.

10. If Mom still refuses, Cedra said that we may have to go and get Mom a Guardian so that we can access the safety deposit box, sell the lake property, and possibly sell Mom's house and land on the interchange. I also have to check out what needs to be done with the CD and shares of oil stock.

PLAN PRIORITIES (done with Cedra's suggestions)

Next 30 days:

1. Meet with the Pastor and solicit his help in convincing Mother to have the paperwork done and move into the Lutheran Home.

   - See if the Faith-based Visiting Nurses from the church can visit Mother weekly and help in her care.

   - Take Mother with the Pastor to go visit the Home and tell her how much it would cost to fix up her house. That she can go the Lutheran Home based on her cash flow and have so much more to do with her friends at the home.

2. Meet with Dr. Throne, show him the things I wrote down about the way she is and see if he'll put her in the hospital and have a cardiologist examine her. Maybe he can get her examined for Alzheimer's, too. Have him call Dr. Creighton to collaborate and tell them both she is drinking and taking her drugs at the same time.

   - What do I do if Mother refuses surgery for her cataracts? How do I handle her if she is blind?

   - With everything that is going on, Mom seems to be going down hill pretty fast. Cedra says this might be something called failure to thrive, and that there is an evaluation for that called the Karnofsky Scale that can tell how much care she needs. Perhaps Dr. Creighton can have that done or get someone to do it.

   - Have him tell Mother that she only has two choices—go to the Lutheran Home or hire someone to live with her full time. Tell her what it would cost to fix the house up right and to pay for someone to live in all the time. She usually responds to issues put in dollars and cents because she lived through the Depression, as she likes to tell us.

3. Ask Mom's attorney to tell me about Mom's will (if he will tell me) and if he won't tell me, ask if he can talk to her about letting me know about it.

4. The idea of a Guardianship is becoming more realistic. Perhaps Dr. Thorne can put Mom in the hospital and then into a nursing home for some rehab while we do a Guardianship.

5. Contact Mother's attorney about preparing the paperwork for the Guardianship or referring us to who can best do it. Cedra said I may need an elder law attorney, especially if we need to go through a Guardianship.

   - How long would it take to do that?

   - If she won't sign paperwork and is a threat to her own well-being what can I do? Aunt Celia has a guardian in her last years.

   - What would I have to do to be Mom's guardian if she won't work with us? I need to ask:
     - How long would that take?
     - What else needs to be done?

- Who else needs to be involved?
- What are the costs?

6. Keep updating the diary and start keeping one for my husband.

7. Keep attending my family caregiver support group.

8. Speak to Mom's postman and ask him if he can please call me immediately if he sees anything unusual about Mom when he delivers the mail. If he says yes, give him my numbers.

9. Put a copy of Mother's healthcare information, doctors, contacts, my numbers, and other important information on the refrigerator at her house in case 911 gets called. Also include Pastor's contact information.

10. Make up and carry a card in my wallet that tells people if I am injured that Mother is home alone, and the authorities need to check on her.

11. Contact the Medic Alert folks and get one of those phone alert systems installed at Mother's house. Have Dr. Throne say that this is not negotiable.

12. Update my brother so that he feels that he has some part to play in Mother's care even though I know he cannot focus on it.

13. Ask Mother if her will includes some financial support for her daughter-in-law and granddaughter with MS.

14. Update this Plan with any new information I get.

Next 60 days:

15. Speak to the handyman about what we absolutely need to repair if Mother has to stay there for the next six months. She really can't be there, but I need to be prepared.

16. Because I am a family caregiver for two people, my health is important. I need to have a complete physical, blood work, Pap smear, etc. I have to be prepared for what may be coming.

17. Make a schedule for how I will deal with all of the family caregiving. Cedra said she will help me with that.

18. Make a Plan for my husband.

19. Find Mother's Ames Funeral parlor paperwork for the pre-need funeral; get a copy from Ames if I have to.

20. Update Mother's Plan with any new information I get.

Next 90 days:

21. Check with the agent on the cottage property and check with Rick on the interchange property.

22. Mother's house is filled with decades of stuff collected from everyone and everywhere. See what she wants done with the furniture and collectibles when she (I hope) goes to live at the Home because everyone in the family has already said they don't want it or need it, and I don't need another stick of anything in my house. Perhaps we should have someone come in and estimate the value of all of it. Be prepared for her to say, "It's all in the will" and not budge.

23. Update Plan with any new information I get.

12.

Additional Resources

Numerous national and local organizations may be able to assist in learning about specific disorders, methods for treatment, support groups, and other critical family caregiving information. Most organizations (although not all) provide toll-free phone numbers and websites. Wherever possible, toll-free numbers and "helplines" are listed, as well as TTY numbers for hearing impaired. Phone numbers are subject to change without notice.

Personal networking with others faced with similar challenges can lead to unexpectedly valuable information. Family caregivers should seek out support groups and grassroots groups in their own neighborhoods.

Additional listings of local chapters of national organizations may be found by referring to directories of local chapters on the national organizations' website.

A word of warning: The Internet is a valuable information source if you use recognized and respected organizations for assistance. Blogs and personal information pages can also be useful with issues; however, take great care in depending on such sources for definitive, reliable information. Some ill-informed and unreliable individuals may have personal conclusions and medical opinions that are worrisome, if not dangerous.

> **Note:** *The information provided was accurate when entered here, but organizations often change both their website addresses and phone numbers. If you find a link or phone number that does not work, please notify the author by email at bkbboots@aol.com.*

FLORIDA RESOURCES

> **Note:** *Similar organizations may exist in any state. Use the agency names given below as key words for searching and create your own list for your state or for the state in which your loved one lives. Add your list to your Plan.*

Agency for Healthcare Administration (agency responsible for licensing healthcare professionals and for licensing and inspecting healthcare facilities), www.ahca.myflorida.com

AHCA Florida Medicaid Reform, www.ahca.myflorida.com/Medicaid/medicaid_reform/index.shtml

Area Agency on Aging by county, www.elderaffairs.state.fl.us/english/aaa.php

Children's Medical Services Network (programs for eligible children with special needs), www.cms-kids.com

Department of Children and Family Services office locations, www.dcf.state.fl.us/ess

Florida Department of Elder Affairs, www.elderaffairs.state.fl.us

Florida Department of Health, www.doh.state.fl.us

Florida Health Finder (consumer information on service providers, insurers, and services throughout state), www.floridahealthfinder.gov

HMO Coverage Sources, www.floridahealthfinder.gov

HMO Report Card, www.floridahealthfinder.gov

Medicaid MediPass, www.ahca.myflorida.com/Medicaid/MediPass/index.shtml

FOR CHILDREN AND TEENS

It is common for children (young people under the age of eighteen) to provide care for siblings and even for adults. And, of course, children and teens are also the recipients of family caregiving. If you know of a resource for children and teens that is not listed here, please send information about it to the following email address: familycaregiver_advocacygroup@aol.com.

ADEAR Center Resources for Children and Teens, www.nia.nih.gov/alzheimers/ alzheimers-disease-information-children-andteens-resource-list

Alzheimer's Association Kids & Teens, www.alz.org/living_with_alzheimers_just_ for_kids_and_teens.asp, 800-272-3900

Alzheimer's Foundation of America (AFA) Teens, http://www.afateens.org, 866-232-8484

NATIONAL RESOURCES

If you have a suggestion for a resource that could be added to this list, please send information about it to the following email address: familycaregiver_advocacygroup@aol.com

Administration on Aging, Elder Care Locator, www.eldercare.gov, 800-677-1116

American Academy on Neurology, neurologist locator, http://patients.aan.com/findaneurologist

American Association for Caregiver Education, www.caregivered.org

American Association for Geriatric Psychiatry, physician finder, www.gmhfonline.org/gmhf/find.asp

American Heart Association (see also "Stroke Connection" in this list), www.americanheart.org, 800-242-8721

American Liver Foundation, www.liverfoundation.org, 212-668-1000

American Lung Association, www.lungusa.org, 800-548-8252

American Parkinson Disease Association, www.apdaparkinson.org, 800-225-2732

ALS Association (Lou Gehrig's Disease), www.alsa.org, 800-782-4747

Arthritis Foundation, www.arthiritis.org

The Association for Frontotemporal Degeneration, www.theaftd.org

Cancer Information Service (division of NIH), cis.nci.nih.gov, 800-422-6237

Cystic Fibrosis Foundation, www.cff.org, 800-344-4823

Depression—Secure Horizons (division of NIMH), www.securehorizons.com, 800-421-4211

Family Caregiver Alliance, www.caregiver.org, 800-445-8106

HIV/AIDS Treatment Information Service (division of National Institutes of Health), www.aidsinfo.nih.gov, 800-448-0440

Huntington's Disease Society of America, www.hdsa.org, 800-345-4372

Leukemia & Lymphoma Society, www.leukemia-lymphoma.org, 800-955-4572

Lewy Body Dementia Association, www.lbda.org
800-539-9767 (toll-free LBD Caregiver Link), 404-935-6444 (national office)
www.lbda.org/content/lbda-scientific-advisory-council (clinic list)
www.lbda.org/content/finding-doctor-diagnose-and-treat-lbd
(doctor locator)

Long Term Care/US Department of Health and Human Services (official site)
http://longtermcare.gov

Lupus Foundation, www.lupus.org, 800-558-0121

Medic Alert Foundation International (registration for illness/medication and location using identification jewelry and/or cards), www.medicalert.org 800-633-4298

Medicaid (Federal agency) and locator for Medicaid state agencies, www.cms.hhs.gov/home/ medicaid.asp

Medicare and Medicare Hotline (Federal hotline), www.medicare.gov, www.cms.hhs.gov/home/medicare.asp, 800-MEDICARE (800-632-4227)

Medline Plus (Federal prescription and medical issues), www.MedlinePlus.gov, www.medlineplus.gov/spanish

Michael J. Fox Foundation for Parkinson's Research, www.michaeljfox.org, 800-708-7644

Muscular Dystrophy Association, www.mda.org, 800-572-1717

National Cancer Institute (division of NIH), www.cancer.gov, 800-422-6237

National Institute on Aging, Alzheimer's Disease Education and Referral (ADEAR) Center (division of NIH), www.nia.nih.gov/alzheimers; for a list of research centers see www.nia.nih.gov/alzheimers/alzheimers-disease-research-centers, 800-438-4380

National Institute of Diabetes & Digestive & Kidney Diseases (division of NIH), www.niddk.nih.gov, 301-496-3583

National Institute of Neurological Disorders and Stroke (division of NIH), www.ninds.nih.gov, 800-352-9424

National Institutes of Health (NIH, Federal agency), www.nih.gov

National Kidney Foundation, www.kidney.org, 800-622-9010

National Mental Health Association, www.nmha.org, 800-969-6642

National Multiple Sclerosis Society, www.nationalMSsociety.org, 800-344-4867

National Osteoporosis Foundation, www.nof.org, 800-223-9994

National Parkinson's Foundation, www.parkinson.org, 800-473-4636

National Stroke Association, www.stroke.org, 800-787-6537

Parkinson's Disease Foundation, www.pdf.org, 800-457-6676

Project Lifesaver International (information on location devices for wanderers), www.projectlifesaver.org, 877-580-5433

Sickle Cell Association of America, www.sicklecelldisease.org, 800-421-8453

Social Security Administration, www.ssa.gov, 800-772-1213 (TTY 800-325-0778).

Spina Bifida Association of America, www.sbaa.org, 800-621-3141

Stroke Connection, American Heart Association, 800-553-6321

United Cerebral Palsy Association, www.ucp.org, 800-872-5827

Veterans Administration, Office of Inspector General
Complaint/Hotline: www.va.gov/oig/hotline/,
Frequently Asked Questions: www.va.gov/oig/hotline/faq.asp
Other contact: vaoighotline@va.gov, 800-488-8244

Appendix

The Family Caregiver Questionnaire

This questionnaire is designed to provide you, the unpaid family caregiver, with a summary of personal information vital to family caregiving decision-making and as a core document for building your Family Caregiving Plan. Spending time now to assemble your family care information will save you time later, both when you prepare your Plan and when you have to make decisions during emergencies.

THE PURPOSE OF THE QUESTIONNAIRE

- Most of us spend our lifetimes looking for documentation we need for our healthcare, legal, and financial paperwork, as well as other family history, contact information, and more.
- Assembling the Questionnaire is a major step forward in getting organized.
- The Questionnaire is the basis for your personal written Plan.

The Questionnaire was originally developed by the American Association for Caregiver Education and the Family Caregiver Advocacy Group (FCAG). FCAG holds the copyright on the Questionnaire and granted permission to use it in this new edition of *The Family Caregiver's Manual*.

- The Plan tells your personal caregiver story, enabling you to better understand what is happening now and what may happen later, as well as how to better prepare.

- You CANNOT prepare an effective Plan until you gather the necessary information; the Questionnaire is an easy-to-use tool that will help you make that happen.

    Note: Users may duplicate the questionnaire to use with others. However, you can purchase additional printed copies of the Questionnaire or a PDF of the form by going to www.caregiverreality.com and going to the Shop.

INSTRUCTIONS FOR COMPLETING THE QUESTIONNAIRE

- If you have been making notes as you worked through the *Manual*, transfer relevant information from your notes to the appropriate place in the Questionnaire.

- **There are two sections to the Questionnaire**—Part 1: The Caregiver and Part 2: The Person Needing Care.

- **The first page of the "Part 2: The Person Needing Care"** includes space for a picture of the person. Having a CURRENT picture can be especially important if you are caring for someone with a medical or cognitive problem that can cause the person to wander. Remember that the appearance of children and the elderly can change very rapidly. You need to update the picture at least once every 6 months.

- **If you are filling in the forms by hand, PLEASE clearly PRINT YOUR RESPONSES SO THAT NO ONE HAS TO DECIPHER WHAT WAS WRITTEN.**

- If you are a family caregiver for a family member, that person's family history and medical history may contain information that is relevant to your own planning for the future—genetic history, the way you were raised, education, financial background, and other factors can affect your health and/or your planning for your personal care.

- **Take your time.** Life, and what happens in life, did not happen in a day. The Questionnaire is a type of life history and you are unlikely to be able to assemble all the needed information in a single sitting or even in a few days.

- **Not everything will be readily available.** You may have to contact agencies and departments to obtain military discharge records, copies of Medicare records, Social Security cards, certified birth certificates, out-of-state doctor and hospital records, family history from relatives, and personal information from friends. BE PATIENT.

- Once you have completed the form, decide who else needs to have all or part of the information included and give them a copy of what they need to know.

- Schedule a date NOW to review the Questionnaire, update of the information, and make any necessary changes in your written Care Plan. A review should be done at least once every 6 months and each time a change in health or another circumstance creates a change.

- Whenever you implement or change care or make a change in any part of the information contained in the Questionnaire, review the entire form to ensure the information is still relevant, update as needed, and keep the information handy along with your up-to-date written Care Plan.

- Finally, **congratulations** on the taking a major step to gaining **family caregiver peace-of-mind.**

Part 1: THE CAREGIVER'S LIST

As a caregiver for another person, it is important that information about you is included in that person's records. Provide the following information about yourself. Also, complete a copy of Part 2 for yourself—you need to plan for you too!

Date Prepared: _____

Your Current Contact Information			
Name			
Street Address			
City/State/Zip		Country	
Cell Phone		Home Phone	
Work Phone		Other Phone	
Primary Email		Other Email	

Your Marital Status
☐ single ☐ married and living with spouse ☐ married and not living with spouse
☐ separated ☐ divorced ☐ domestic partnership ☐ other: _____

Relationship to the Person Requiring Care	
Type of relationship	
Do you live with this person? ☐ Yes ☐ No	
Does this make you a local (live within 1 hour driving distance) or long distance caregiver (travel more than an hour to visit)? _____	

Your Family Caregiver Responsibilities
Are you a decision maker, a hands-on caregiver, or both?

If you are currently providing care, how long have you been providing care?

What is your expectation as to how long you may be required to continue to provide care for this person?

Who assists you in providing care?

Name		Phone	
Address			
Relationship to You		Relationship to Person Needing Care	

In what ways does this person assist you?

Name		Phone	
Address			
Relationship to You		Relationship to Person Needing Care	

In what ways does this person assist you?

What tasks do you perform now?

What tasks do you expect to perform in the near term and in the future? (If you have not done so, complete the scale "Defining Yourself as a Family Caregiver.")

How would you describe your emotional state? Attitude? Stress level?
(If you have not done so already, complete and list your scores for the
"Problem-Solving Attitude" and "Caregiver Stress" checklists.)

Your Goals
(attach additional pages if necessary)

List your current goals as a family caregiver.

List your current goals for your personal well-being.

**List what you feel are your physical, financial, and emotional
limitations in providing care for your loved one.**

What are your other concerns (family issues, work issues, social issues, other)?

**Every caregiver should complete a copy of Part 2 for him/herself.
It is also useful to prepare similar forms for every family member.**

We all need to plan for the future.

Part 2: THE PERSON NEEDING CARE NOW OR IN THE FUTURE

Remember: Some information may not apply. If so, leave blank. However, fill in as many spaces as possible. If necessary, add pages, but be sure to identify what section the answers apply to (e.g., Personal Data, Section I).

Date Prepared: _____

Name of Person Needing Care	
Nickname Person Answers to	

Does this person have a cognitive or mental health problem that impairs his/her ability to understand questions or instructions?   ☐ No   ☐ Yes

If yes, indicate the type of impairment:

Does this person currently have a physical/health problem or a disability that impairs his/her ability to walk, see, or perform physically?   ☐ No   ☐ Yes

If yes, indicate the type of impairment:

PERSONAL DATA

Section I. KEY INFORMATION

Current, full-face photo in color; face image is at least 2½ inches high

     Date Taken: _____

Keep **current** full-face and full-height photos that can be used to identify individual. Where are these photos kept? _____

Are digital copies available? ☐ No   ☐ Yes

Date Taken: _____

Location of the digital file: _____

Birth Date	Age	Height	Weight	Blood Type

Birthmarks/Scars:

Person's Home Address:

Street	

City		State		Zip	

Person's Home Phone Number	

Person's Email Address	

Names of Streets at Closest Main Intersection:

Closest Hospital	
Street Address	
Hospital Phone Number	
Emergency Room Number	

Most recent date person was in this hospital and reason:

Identification document(s)—Check all that apply and indicate location

☐ **Driver's License** # _____ State Issued by: _____

   Location: _____ Renewal Date: _____

☐ **State approved identification card** # _____

   Location: _____

☐ **Residence status document** Type: _____

   Location: _____

☐ **Passport** Issuing Country: _____ Document #: _____

   Location: _____ Renewal Date: _____

☐ **Other**—provide type, issuing agency, number _____

   _____

   _____

   Which of identification does person always carry? Where is it carried?

Vital Insurance and Benefit Numbers

Primary Healthcare Insurance

Provider Name	
Individual or Group Policy Number	
Contact Number	
Social Security Number	
Medicare Number	
Medicaid Number	
Veterans Identification Number	

Language	
Primary Language Spoken	
Level of Usage ☐ Fluent ☐ Needs assistance	Is an interpreter required? ☐ No ☐ Yes
If an interpreter is required, it is useful to identify in advance a person who can perform this task to ensure the language/dialect used is appropriate.	
Interpreter's Name	
Contact Number	
Relationship to person needing care	

Marital Status	
☐ single ☐ married and living with spouse ☐ married and not living with spouse ☐ separated ☐ divorced ☐ domestic partnership ☐ other:_____	
If person is married, but not living with his/her spouse, where does his/her spouse live?	

Emergency Contact Information	
Name of Person	
Relationship to Person Needing Care	
Cell Phone		Home Phone	
Business Phone		Personal Email	
Is this person a designated power of attorney? ☐ No ☐ Yes	Is the person the designated healthcare surrogate? ☐ No ☐ Yes
Does physician/hospital/other medical professional have copy of designation documents? ☐ No ☐ Yes	

Does the person have a professional care planning advisor, social worker, geriatric case manager, or other professional who assists with planning or implementing care? If so, provide the requested information.

Name of Person	

Cell Phone		Other Phone	

Email	

How long has this person been working with the individual needing care?	

What are this person's qualifications and how does his/her professional experience support the needs of the person needing care?

Healthcare Provider List		
Type	**Name**	**Contact Number**
Primary Care Physician		
Specialist (give type)		
Specialist (give type)		
Other (give type)		
Other (give type)		
Pharmacist (give location of pharmacy here)		

Section II. HEALTH INSURANCE
List and describe all policies.

Provider name	
Policy holder ID number	
Type of insurance (e.g., health, disability, long-term care)	
Fees for service(s) ☐ No ☐ Yes	Preapprovals Required For:
Claims support number	

Provider name	
Policy holder ID number	
Type of insurance (e.g., health, disability, long-term care)	
Fees for service(s) ☐ No ☐ Yes	Preapprovals Required For:
Claims support number	

Provider name	
Policy holder ID number	
Type of insurance (e.g., health, disability, long-term care)	
Fees for service(s) ☐ No ☐ Yes	Preapprovals Required For:
Claims support number	

Provider name	
Policy holder ID number	
Type of insurance (e.g., health, disability, long-term care)	
Fees for service(s) ☐ No ☐ Yes	Preapprovals Required For:
Claims support number	

If necessary, list additional policies on a separate sheet. Provide all requested information.

Section III. MILTARY SERVICE HISTORY & VETERANS BENEFITS

Veteran's serial number	
Branch of service	
Highest rank attained	
Enlistment date	
Discharge date	
Place (base, city, state, etc.) discharged	
Served during time of combat? ☐ No ☐ Yes	If yes, where? _____ When? _____
Wounded in combat? ☐ No ☐ Yes If yes, describe.	
Currently receiving VA benefits? ☐ No ☐ Yes If yes, what types?	
Location of military records	

Section IV. MEDICAL CARE

Manages own medicines, makes and keeps doctor appointments ☐ No ☐ Yes

If no, how are these activities handled?

Gets regular preventive care for health conditions ☐ No ☐ Yes

If no, why not?

Last Physical	Date done		Where given	
Done by			Telephone	

Tests done (blood, scans, x-rays, EKG, urinalysis, cognitive function tests, other):

Results/major findings:

Recommended post-exam care or follow-up, date, time, location:

In the past 12 months, has this person experienced one or more health-related incidents, such as a serious fall, new chronic condition, major change in existing chronic condition? If so, describe the event and the changes that it has caused.

How often does the person visit physicians or healthcare providers? Why? Provide name of provider, frequency of visit, and reason.

Section V. CAPABILITIES & OTHER ISSUES			
Indicate whether person does things always, sometimes, or never.			
Task	Always	Sometimes	Never
Does own shopping for groceries and other items (including clothes)			
Prepares own meals			
Handles personal hygiene needs (bathing, hair care, dressing, etc.)			
Manages own finances (pays bills, balances checkbook, etc.)			
Does housekeeping chores and does/does not require assistance			
Drives or otherwise manages personal transportation needs; has current license tags, driver's license, and vehicle insurance			
Has chronic conditions; list all (e.g., high blood pressure, arthritis, diabetes, etc.)			
Uses assistive devices (e.g., wheelchair, walker, cane, hearing aid, glasses, dentures, etc.)			
Is occasionally confused or forgetful			
Seems moody or depressed			
Takes good care of him/herself (e.g., maintains good hygiene, personal appearance, etc.)			
Is beginning to rely more on others			

Other Issues
Currently smokes? ☐ No ☐ Yes If yes, describe effects.
Smoked in the past? ☐ No ☐ Yes If yes, describe effects.
Has trouble hearing? ☐ No ☐ Yes If yes, describe effects.
Uses a hearing aid? ☐ No ☐ Yes If yes, describe effects.
Has impaired vision? ☐ No ☐ Yes If yes, list type of impairment (e.g., glaucoma, macular degeneration, cataracts, etc.) and describe effects.

Wears glasses? ☐ No ☐ Yes	Wears contacts? ☐ No ☐ Yes

If yes, why does person wear corrective lenses? ☐ Nearsighted ☐ Farsighted ☐ Other: _____
Had corrective eye surgery? ☐ No ☐ Yes If yes, give type and describe effects.

Wears dentures? ☐ No   ☐ Yes   If yes, how old are they? Do they fit well?

Has artificial limb or other prosthesis? ☐ No   ☐ Yes   If yes, describe.

Has insulin pump? ☐ No   ☐ Yes   If yes, when inserted? _____

Has pacemaker? ☐ No   ☐ Yes   If yes, when inserted? _____

Has pain pump? ☐ No   ☐ Yes   If yes, when inserted? _____

Being tube fed? ☐ No   ☐ Yes   If yes, when inserted? _____
Is there a central line? ☐ No   ☐ Yes

Needs oxygen? ☐ No   ☐ Yes   If yes, check how received: ☐ Home Pump
☐ Portable Pump   ☐ Other method: _____

Currently in dialysis? ☐ No   ☐ Yes   If yes, treatment began _____

Frequency: _____   Location: _____

How does person travel to location? _____

Weight
Ever diagnosed as overweight? ☐ No ☐ Yes If yes, what was reason, if known?
Ever diagnosed as underweight? ☐ No ☐ Yes If yes, what was reason, if known?
Recently gained weight? ☐ No ☐ Yes If yes, what was reason, if known?
Recently lost weight? ☐ No ☐ Yes If yes, what was reason, if known?
Feels fatigue/weakness? ☐ No ☐ Yes If yes, what was reason, if known?

Section VI. FAMILY CAREGIVER RESPONSIBILITIES

A person needing care may also be a family caregiver, which may mean that you have to plan for alternative family caregivers for one or more loved ones he/she is caring for when the person is unable to provide care for that loved one.

Person needing care is what relationship to the person(s) being cared for?

Name of person (list all)	Adult or child?	Reason for care (mental/physical illness, short term, chronic, seriousness, etc.)

How long has the person been providing care?		
Describe family caregiving situation (e.g., type of care, location of care, etc.):		
Is someone assisting in providing care? If so, provide the following information.		

		Phone Number	
Assistant's Name		Phone Number	
Relationship to person giving care		Relationship to people receiving care	

Does the person you are planning care for express concerns over his/her ability to be a family caregiver? ☐ No   ☐ Yes If yes, describe.

Section VII. LIFESTYLE INFORMATION

Work History

Retired?　☐ No　☐ Yes　If yes, when? _____　At what age? _____

Did person retire because of health issues?　☐ No　☐ Yes　If yes, explain.

Current Occupation (if working)

Title	Hours worked _____	Perception of stress ☐ high ☐ moderate ☐ low
	Years Worked _____	
Description of work done		Level of activity active, semi-active, inactive

Hazardous occupation (mining, exposure to asbestos, etc.)?
☐ No　☐ Yes　If yes, describe hazard.

Previous Occupation

Title	Hours worked _____	Perception of stress ☐ high ☐ moderate ☐ low
	Years Worked _____	
Description of work done		Level of activity active, semi-active, inactive

Hazardous occupation (mining, exposure to asbestos, etc.)?
☐ No　☐ Yes　If yes, describe hazard.

Is the person currently volunteering his/her time? If so, indicate where, type of service, number of hours worked, and how long has been volunteering.

Educational Background

Educational Level (Give school name if possible)	Graduated?		Location
	Yes	No	
Elementary School			
Junior High School			
High School			
Community College (2-year)			
College (4-year)			
Graduate School			

Does person currently attend classes? ☐ No ☐ Yes If yes, describe.

Living Children (if any)

Name	Sex	Age	Lives in same home?		Lives in same city?		Lives elsewhere? Give city/state/etc.
			Yes	No	Yes	No	

If you need additional space to list individuals, attach additional pages. Include same information.			
Describe racial heritage of children (which can influence decision-making).			
Which of these children currently assists with family care for person needing care? And what do they do?			

LIVING SITUATION			

Lives alone? ☐ Yes   ☐ No   If no, list competent individuals he/she lives with below.

Name		Relationship to person	
Cell phone		Work phone	
Primary email		Other email	
Name		Relationship to person	
Cell phone		Work phone	
Primary email		Other email	
Name		Relationship to person	
Cell phone		Work phone	
Primary email		Other email	

If the person lives alone and he/she has a critical medical condition, does he/she have a Life Alert or similar emergency alert product?   ☐ Yes   ☐ No

If no, consideration should be given to obtaining one.

Type of Housing

Safety/Security/Condition Checklist

When you have completed the checklist on the residence, attach a copy of that Checklist to this form so that it can be referred to as needed when you complete the form, develop the Plan, and update in the future.

Living arrangements—CHECK BOXES FOR ALL THAT APPLY.

☐ **Owns home**
　☐ single family ☐ apartment ☐ condominium ☐ duplex ☐ multiplex

☐ **Rents**
　☐ single family ☐ apartment ☐ condominium ☐ duplex ☐ multiplex

☐ **Planned community**
　☐ single family ☐ apartment ☐ condominium ☐ duplex ☐ multiplex

☐ **Special needs residence**
　☐ house ☐ apartment ☐ group home

☐ **Assisted living facility**
　☐ single space ☐ shared space/how many share space? _____

☐ **Nursing home**
　☐ single space ☐ shared space/how many share space? _____

☐ **Life community** (different levels of care/independent to nursing care provided)
　What level of care does person reside in? _____
　☐ single space ☐ shared space/ how many share space? _____

Number of floors		**Lives on what floor if more than one floor in residence?**	

If more than one floor, must upper floors be accessed only on the outside of building?
☐ No ☐ Yes

If yes, how are upper floors accessed?
☐ By exterior elevator ☐ By exterior stairs between floors ☐ By both methods

If more than one floor in residence, how are floors accessed **in the interior** of the residence? ☐ By elevator ☐ By stairs between floors ☐ By both methods

Number of exterior access doors to residence _____

　Locations: _____

How are the doors opened?
　☐ Key/key care ☐ Security code ☐ By staff from inside

Is facility (or floor) a secure facility (or floor)? This means, are residents living in a controlled environment where their ability to leave unaccompanied by staff is limited due to dementia or another cognitive or mental health issue. ☐ No ☐ Yes

Reason it is secured: _____

If yes, how doors are opened?
☐ Key/key card ☐ Security code must be entered on a keypad
☐ Locked and opened only by staff from inside ☐ No door security provided

Bedrooms and Bathrooms		
Floor	**1st Floor**	**Upper Floors**
Number of bedrooms		
Number of bedrooms next to baths		
Number of half baths		
Number of full baths		
Number of baths with shower/tub combination		
Number of baths with separate shower		
Bathrooms are ADA compliant and disabled-ready (doors wide enough for wheelchair, grab bars installed, etc.)	☐ Yes ☐ No	☐ Yes ☐ No
Is there a walk-in shower?	☐ Yes ☐ No	☐ Yes ☐ No

Considering the current condition of the person needing care, is the residence in proper condition for occupancy, adapted as needed to be safe, and in all other ways an appropriate place for the person to reside? ☐ Yes ☐ No

If the answer is "NO," summarize the modifications that are necessary in order to make it an appropriate residence. Add additional page(s) if needed.

If the residence is a private home, what is the estimated cost for making modifications that have to be made by a professional? $_____

How long will it take to make required modifications to the residence?

If the residence is a care facility, are plans in place to modify the care facility to make it more appropriate? ☐ No ☐ Yes   If yes, what is the administration's plan for making necessary changes and how long will the project take?

If the home is a private residence, is there room for live-in help (private room and bath, for example)? ☐ No ☐ Yes

If yes, where is that room and bath located in relationship to the room of the person needing care?

Transportation

Drives? ☐ No ☐ Yes   If yes, list issuing state and renewal date of driver's license.

State _____ Renewal date _____

Has own car? ☐ No ☐ Yes   If yes, describe condition of car and any special equipment (such as adaptation for disability).

If the person drives, how often does this person drive him/herself to and from places?
☐ always ☐ most of the time ☐ sometimes ☐ never

Has the person been issued a handicapped parking sticker? ☐ No ☐ Yes If yes:

▪ The sticker is ☐ permanent ☐ temporary

▪ If the sticker is a temporary sticker, when does temporary period end? _____

If the person owns one or more vehicles, but no longer drives, are plans in place for disposing of the vehicles he/she owns? ☐ No ☐ Yes
If no, why not?

If yes, how and within what time frame?

If the person does not drive at all or uses other forms of transportation, indicate type of transportation used.

☐ Drives self in own car   How often: _____
☐ Drives self in rental car   How often: _____
☐ Uses taxi cab   How often: _____
☐ Uses public bus   How often: _____
☐ Uses local in-city train   How often: _____
☐ Uses subway   How often: _____
☐ Family caregiver (person filling out this form) drives him/her
      How often: _____
☐ Family member other than person filling out the form drives him/her
      How often: _____
      Which family member(s): _____
☐ Friend or neighbor provides transportation   How often: _____
☐ Paid caregiver drives him/her in family vehicle   How often: _____
☐ Paid caregiver drives him/her in paid caregiver's car   How often: _____
☐ Uses nonmedical group bus ride   How often: _____
☐ Uses disabled or medical transport   How often: _____
☐ Uses senior transportation   How often: _____

If the person does not use disabled, medical, or senior transportation, is it available?
☐ No   ☐ Yes   If yes, what type?

Why doesn't the person use one of these options?

If the person does not use public transportation, why not?

NUTRITION AND DINING HABITS

Dietary restrictions?   ☐ No   ☐ Yes   If yes, describe.

Favorite foods?   ☐ No   ☐ Yes   If yes, are favorites off limits because of dietary restrictions?

Prepares own meals at home?   ☐ Yes   ☐ No   If no, how are meals provided and what is the name person or service that provides the meals?

At home, dines alone or with someone?   ☐ Alone
☐ With someone   If with someone, who dines with person most often?

Eats out?   ☐ No   ☐ Yes   If yes, how often and where (restaurant, congregate meal site for seniors and its location, other person's home)?

Average cost per month for restaurant/eat-out meals if pays personally: $_____
Is this expense listed in the person's budget plan?   ☐ No   ☐ Yes

PHYSICAL ACTIVITY
Does the person engage in physical activity? ☐ No ☐ Yes
If no, are plans in place to start exercising? ☐ No ☐ Yes
If engages in physical activity, does he/she get 30 minutes or more of vigorous exercise 3 or more times a week? ☐ No ☐ Yes
If yes, check off the activities the person engages in. ☐ walking ☐ biking ☐ swimming ☐ jogging ☐ aerobics ☐ strength exercises ☐ yoga ☐ chair exercises ☐ strength exercises ☐ yardwork ☐ mowing lawn ☐ household chores ☐ Other: _____
Exercises at home? ☐ No ☐ Yes Goes to a gym or exercise program (e.g., YMCA, senior center, yoga class) outside of home? ☐ No ☐ Yes

SOCIAL, CULTURAL, OTHER ACTIVITIES List and indicate how often engages in interest or activity.
List interests (music, art, history, etc.).
List hobbies.
List organizations and social groups belongs to and attends.
Describe religious activities.
Other

PETS			
Type	Name	Age	ID chip in place? Yes or No

Provide name and contact information for veterinarian.

Name, location, and phone number for the nearest boarding kennel or name of person who will provide care in an emergency.

Can the person properly care for pets now without assistance? ☐ Yes   ☐ No
If no, how are pets going to be cared for now? In the future?

If the person became permanently unable to care for his/her pet(s), what are the arrangements for finding the pets a new home?

Monthly cost of food and pet care: $_____
Is this expense included in the person's budget? ☐ Yes   ☐ No If no, add to budget.

Having trouble locating all the information you need?

Remember: Patience is the key in family caregiving and when completing this form.

Also, remember: Having a plan makes things work better—

what's your plan for locating the missing information?

Section VIII: MEDICAL HISTORY

FAMILY MEDICAL HISTORY

Note: A thorough family medical history may be important in diagnosing illnesses.

- List information for the following individuals if possible: father, mother, grandfather and grandmother on father's side, grandfather and grandmother on mother's side, mother's and father's siblings (person's aunts and uncles), person's siblings, and person's children.

- Add pages if necessary; clearly identify relationships if you add pages.

- Age at death, cause of death, ethnicity, health conditions—all may provide information that helps a medical professional understand a person's health issues.

- If the person was adopted and does not have information on blood relatives, leave this section on blood-related parents, grandparents, aunts, uncles, and siblings blank.

Relationship to Person (enter name)	Birth Year	Age if living	Age at death	Year of death	Current health conditions or cause of death (list major chronic conditions, e.g., dementia, heart disease)
Father, Mother, Grandparents					
Father _____ Ethnic Origin: _____					
Mother _____ Ethnic Origin: _____					
Father's Mother _____ Ethnic Origin: _____					
Father's Father _____ Ethnic Origin: _____					
Mother's Mother _____ Ethnic Origin: _____					
Mother's Father _____ Ethnic Origin: _____					

Relationship to Person (enter name)	Birth Year	Age if living	Age at death	Year of death	Current health conditions or cause of death (list major chronic conditions, e.g., dementia, heart disease)
Father's Siblings (circle male/female—M or F)					
M F Name					
M F Name					
M F Name					
M F Name					
M F Name					
Mother's Siblings (circle male/female—M or F)					
M F Name					
M F Name					
M F Name					
M F Name					
M F Name					
Person's Siblings (circle male/female—M or F)					
M F Name					
M F Name					

Relationship to Person (enter name)	Birth Year	Age if living	Age at death	Year of death	Current health conditions or cause of death (list major chronic conditions, e.g., dementia, heart disease)
M F Name					
M F Name					
M F Name					
Person's Children (circle male/female—M or F)					
M F Name					
M F Name					
M F Name					
M F Name					
M F Name					

Are there any conditions on either side of the person's blood-related family that appear to indicate a pattern of genetic/inheritable diseases? If so, describe them.

PERSON'S ALLERGIES

Does the person have allergies?

☐ Do not know.
☐ No   If no, proceed to next section.
☐ Yes   If yes, fill out this section.

Whether you answered "No" or "Yes," has the person <u>actually been tested</u> to determine allergies?

☐ Yes   If yes, how long ago?   _____
☐ No

If the answer is "No," are there plans to have testing done?   ☐ No   ☐ Yes   If yes, when will the testing be done?

Note: Allergies can lead to skin and lung infections and other medical issues that can impair function. Some people are sufficiently allergic to a substance that their reactions can lead to death. If the person needing care has not been tested, it is suggested that he/she visit an allergist for testing.

List **all allergies to foods, cosmetics, detergents, etc.** and describe the person's reactions.

MEDICATIONS (INCLUDING VITAMINS) <u>NOT TO BE TAKEN</u>.

Prescription medications (by brand name taken or by generic name if taken as generic)	
Over-the-counter	
Homeopathic	
Herbal	
Alternative	

DEMENTIA
If the person has been diagnosed as having a form of dementia, please provide information requested below.
When was this diagnosis made (include year)?
Who made the diagnosis (e.g., family physician, neurologist specializing in dementia and cognitive disorders, psychologist, psychiatrist, a team of medical and other specialists specializing in cognitive disorder diagnosis)?
What type of dementia (e.g., frontotemporal lobe, Alzheimer's disease) was diagnosed and what was the stage of disease when the person was tested?
Have you noticed a progression of symptoms in the last 12 months? If so, describe.

Medications Specifically Taken for Dementia			
Medication Name	**Dosage**	**Frequency Taken**	**Administered by self or others?**
			☐ By self ☐ By_____
			☐ By self ☐ By_____
			☐ By self ☐ By_____
			☐ By self ☐ By_____

Is the person participating in a drug-related research study? ☐ No   ☐ Yes

If yes, when did his/her participation begin? _____
If yes, has his/her medication been altered as part of the study? ☐ No   ☐ Yes
If his/her medication has been altered, in what way has it been altered?

Have you noticed any negative side effects since the alteration? If so, please discuss those effects with the research staff as soon as possible.

Describe the behavior and other issues shown by person at this time.

ADDITIONAL CONDITIONS AND MEDICATIONS TAKEN

- **Include prescription drugs; over-the-counter, homeopathic, alternative, and herbal products; vitamins.**
- **A person has a condition even if it is under control using medication.** List that condition and say it is under control (e.g., if a person takes medication to keep blood pressure down and the medication works, the person still has high blood pressure).

Condition	Medication Name	Dosage	Frequency	Administered by self or others?
Sleeplessness				☐ By self ☐ By_____
Arthritis				☐ By self ☐ By_____
Pain				☐ By self ☐ By_____
				☐ By self ☐ By_____
High Blood Pressure				☐ By self ☐ By_____
				☐ By self ☐ By_____

High cholesterol				☐ By self ☐ By_____
				☐ By self ☐ By_____
Fluid/Edema				☐ By self ☐ By_____
				☐ By self ☐ By_____
Cardiac (List all.)				☐ By self ☐ By_____
				☐ By self ☐ By_____
				☐ By self ☐ By_____
Diabetes (List type.)				☐ By self ☐ By_____
Depression				☐ By self ☐ By_____
				☐ By self ☐ By_____
Stress				☐ By self ☐ By_____
Dementia (described under Medical History)				☐ By self ☐ By_____
				☐ By self ☐ By_____
Other mental health issue (List type.)				☐ By self ☐ By_____
				☐ By self ☐ By_____
				☐ By self ☐ By_____

Vitamin deficiency (List type.)				☐ By self ☐ By_____
				☐ By self ☐ By_____
Preventive vitamin therapy				☐ By self ☐ By_____
Thyroid condition (List type.)				☐ By self ☐ By_____
Stomach condition (List type.)				☐ By self ☐ By_____
Eye condition (List type.)				☐ By self ☐ By_____
List any others below				
				☐ By self ☐ By_____
				☐ By self ☐ By_____
				☐ By self ☐ By_____
				☐ By self ☐ By_____
				☐ By self ☐ By_____
More conditions? Add pages if necessary.				

VACCINATIONS				
Vaccination Name	Date First Given	If any reaction, note here.	Most Recent Booster Given	If any reaction, note here.
Anthrax				
Diphtheria-Tetanus				
Hepatitis A				
Hepatitis B				
Herpes Zoster (Shingles)				
Human Papillomavirus (HPV)				
Japanese Encephalitis				
Measles				
Mumps				
Rubella				
Pneumococcal—Old style single shot				
Pneumococcal—New style (1 shot followed by another 6 months later)				
Polio				
Rabies				

Rotavirus	.			
Typhoid				
Smallpox				
Yellow Fever				

Other Vaccinations				

Has Person for any reason ever traveled in Africa, Mid-East or Far East? If so, he/she may have received vaccinations not listed above. If possible, enter that information below.

Vaccination Name	Date Given	Traveled to what location? For how long?

Seasonal Flu Vaccine
Date of Last Vaccination: _____
Describe any reactions:

If the person does NOT take seasonal influenza vaccinations, why not?

H1N1 (indicate drops or shot)
Date of Last Vaccination: _____
Describe any reactions:

If the person does NOT take H1N1 vaccinations, why not?

SURGICAL HISTORY (list most recent surgery first)			
Date	**Hospital**	**Surgeon**	**Kind of Surgery**
More surgeries? Add pages.			

NON-SURGICAL HOSPITAL, SKILLED NURSING FACILITY STAYS (list most recent surgery first)			
Date	Facility	Physician	Reason for Stay
More facility stays? Add pages.			

PERSON'S HISTORY OF ILLNESS		
Major Illness	When?	Please describe course of illness and its treatment; also describe any aftereffects being experienced now.
Major Childhood Illness		
Cancer		
Other		
Other		
Other		
More information? Add pages.		

PERSON'S ONGOING ILLNESSES OR DISABILITIES		
If the subject person has a chronic illness, please describe below.		
Illness/Disability	Year Began	Please describe course of illness and its treatment.
Alzheimer's disease or another cognitive disorder (please name)		
Parkinson's disease		
Kidney disease		
Cancer (give type)		
More information? Add pages		

Additional Comments Regarding Medical History/Health:

FINANCIAL AND LEGAL INFORMATION

Section I: FINANCIAL AND LEGAL ADVISORS

Type of Advisor	Name	Phone Number	Specific Work Done
Attorney			
Accountant			
Financial Planner			
Insurance Agent			
Broker			

Section II: LEGAL DOCUMENTS

Document	Dated	Prepared by	Location	Designee
Will				
Living will				
Trusts, revocable, irrevocable, living, etc.				
Healthcare surrogate				
Durable Power of Attorney (business only)				
Durable Power of Attorney with medical authorization				

Missing Documents

If a document from the list has not been prepared, what plans are being made to prepare one? When will this be done and what professional will assist in the process?

Section III: PERSONAL PAPERS

List the following personal papers, including identification/account numbers or description, issuing agency, and location where copies are stored. Note: It is advisable to scan these records into a digital format and store the digital copies in a safe place.

Document	ID/Account # if any or description	Issuing Agency	Location where person's copy is stored
Birth certificate			
Passport			
Adoption papers			
Naturalization papers			
Official state picture identification			
Marriage certificate(s)			
Divorce decree(s)			
Social Security card			
Social Security benefit records			
Medicaid card			
VA and military records			

Warranties and Service Contracts		
Provider	**What Is Covered**	**Contact Number**

Vehicle Titles					
Make/Model	**Year**	**Vehicle Identification Number (VIN)**	**Owned? Leased?**	**If leased, date expires**	**Location of vehicle and title**

Section IV: TAX RECORDS		
Type	**Years**	**Location**
Federal		
State		
City		
Property/Similar Taxes		

Section V: PRE-NEED FUNERAL PLANS

- Provide the following information for each plan.
- Attach an additional sheet <u>if there is more than one plan</u> or you need to provide additional information.

Funeral Home		Phone	
Prepaid Plan ☐ No ☐ Yes		Irrevocable? ☐ No ☐ Yes	Payout Amount:
Copy of agreement located where?		Cemetery deeds located where?	

If there is no prepaid plan, describe plans for paying when need arises.

Section VI: CREDIT CARDS

Name of Card	Account Number	Account PIN Password	Location of Card

Section VII: CHECKING/SAVINGS/BANKING			
CHECKING ACCOUNTS AND DEBIT CARDS			
Bank Name/Branch Location	**Website**	**Account Number/ PIN**	**Location of Check/ Passbook**
SAVINGS ACCOUNTS			
Bank Name/Branch Location	**Website**	**Account Number/ PIN**	**Location of Check/ Passbook**
Section VIII: BILL PAYMENT			
Company			
Mailing Address			
Customer Service Number			
Account Number			
Website			
User Name/Password			

Auto pay ☐ No ☐ Yes				
Minimum Payment				
Date due or date auto pay made				
If auto pay, payment made through which account?				
Where are charge and payment records kept?				

- Most companies have security questions for on-line account management. If security questions are associated with one or all of the above accounts, note the questions and answers by account on a separate page.

- If there are additional accounts, attach additional pages and provide the same information as above.

Section IX: INVESTMENTS

- If you can manage any of the following categories of investments on-line, remember that most banks, brokerage companies, pension management companies, etc., have security questions for on-line account management. If security questions are associated with one or all of the above accounts, note the questions and answers by account on a separate page.

- If needed, attach additional pages and provide the information listed for each category.

CERTIFICATES OF DEPOSIT

Bank				
Branch				
Customer Service Number				
Account Number				
Website				

User Name/ Password				
Certificate Value				
Location of Certificates				
BROKERAGE ACCOUNTS				
Company				
Broker's Name				
Customer Service Number				
Account Number				
Account Type				
Website				
User Name/ Password				
STOCKS AND BONDS NOT HELD IN BROKERAGE ACCOUNTS				
Company				
Contact Person				
Customer Service Number				
Account Number				
Account Type				

Website				
User Name/ Password				
Location of Share Certificates				
ANNUNITIES				
Company				
Contact Person				
Customer Service Number				
Account Number				
Account Type				
Website				
User Name/ Password				
Location of Policy Copy				

**ARE YOU KEEPING A RUNNING TOTAL
OF THE VALUE OF INVESTMENTS AND OTHER ASSETS?**

IRA(S) AND SIMILAR RETIREMENT FUNDS			
Company			
Contact Person			
Customer Service Number			
Account Number			
Account Type			
Website			
User Name/ Password			
Location of Plan Information			
PENSION PLANS			
Company			
Contact Person			
Customer Service Number			
Account Number			
Account Type			
Website			
User Name/ Password			
Location of Plan Certificate			

Section X: PROPERTY RECORDS

If you rent out a property, note the following:

- If self managing, attach a separate piece of paper listing tenants' names and units (if more than one residential unit), contact information, and renewal date of lease.
- If a management company, on a separate piece of paper provide contact information, monthly fee, length of contract, and location of contract.

Property Address		Date Purchased	
Mortgage Holder		Payment Amount/ Due Date	
Customer Service No.		Account Number	
Website		User Name/ Password	
Special Conditions (e.g., balloon payment, life tenant)			
Rented out? ☐ No ☐ Yes	If yes, monthly income	Total monthly expenses	Location of Lease

Property Address			
Mortgage Holder		Payment Amount/ Due Date	
Customer Service No.		Account Number	
Website		User Name/ Password	
Special Conditions (e.g., balloon payment, life tenant)			
Rented out? ☐ No ☐ Yes	If yes, monthly income	Total monthly expenses	Location of Lease
Additional Information:			

Section XI: INSURANCE				
HEALTH AND HEALTH RELATED INSURANCE IS LISTED IN SECTION II.				
Type	**Life**	**Property**	**Liability**	**Homeowners/ Renters**
Provider				
Customer Service Number				
Policy Number or ID				
Benefit Amount				
Website				
User Name & Password				
Location of Policy				
Type	**Vehicle**			
Provider				
Customer Service Number				
Policy Number or ID				
Benefit Amount				
Website				
User Name & Password				
Location of Policy				

Section XII: INVENTORY

- **The content of an inventory depends on the property you are listing—so, there is no standardized format.**
- **Prepare an inventory of property and attach it to this document. Include the following information:**
  - Description of the item
  - Estimated value
  - Date of purchase and/or installation
  - Location of item
  - Copy of purchase receipt or purchase contract with payment history
  - Estimated value or documentation of an evaluation of condition and current value prepared by a professional
  - A photo or a video recording
  - It is advisable to create a computer file of this information and give another hard copy to at least one other person.

Once the inventory is complete, total the value of all items and determine whether the inventoried items constitute a countable asset in planning.

Review the level of insurance on inventoried items (too little? too much?) and determine whether insurance coverage should be adjusted. A consideration: Full coverage may be too costly in relation to the person's income. What are the options for coverage?

TIP: It is easier to add new items to an inventory as they are acquired or to remove them as they are disposed of instead of trying to update the inventory only occasionally.

Section XIII: DOCUMENT & PROPERTY STORAGE NOT LISTED ABOVE

SAFETY DEPOSIT BOXES

Bank/Address	Box Number	Key Location	Contents

SAFES		
Location	**Location of Key or Combination**	**Contents**

COMPUTERIZED RECORDS	
Record Description or Title	**Computer Used, Drive Name, Folder Name, File Name**

If a computer, disk drive, storage disk, folder, or file is password protected, list that information under the "computer used" column as part of the locator information.

STORAGE UNITS					
Company Name	Address	Unit Number	Gate Password	Key or Combination Location	Contents of Unit (Attach inventory if necessary)

Section XIV: WEBSITES REGULARLY USED TO ANSWER IMPORTANT QUESTIONS			
Site Name	URL	User Name	Password

XV. Other Information

Is there **other information** about the person's life history, lifestyle, health, legal matters, etc., that could be useful? Enter here or add additional pages.

Does the person have an online personal health record? ☐ No ☐ Yes
If yes, how is it accessed (e.g., website, user name, password)?

What is the location of prior x-rays, scans, blood tests that may be in your loved one's possession?

INCOME AND EXPENSES—The Budget

Carefully examining **MONTHLY income and expenses** at the outset provides the best chance of containing expenses, stretching funds over the long-term, and preserving assets. List the items below that apply. Include most recent or monthly average dollar amounts (estimate where necessary).

Note: *It is advisable to create files for each of the items listed in the Income and Expenses sections. In that file, retain award letters (such as the annual notice of Social Security payment amounts), 1099 forms, investment statements. Also retain copies of bills by type of bill (e.g., utility bills, mortgage statements).*

Also consider scanning and retaining these records in digital form, being sure to store them in a secure location.

INCOME

Income Item	Monthly	Annual
Salary/wages (by each employer)		
Social Security		
Pension(s)		

Annuities		
Stock Dividends		
IRAs		
Bonds		
Mutual Funds		
Rental Property Income (by property)		
Other Income		

Total this income.		

EXPENSES		
Expense Item **(Note: If renovations or equipment replacements** **are anticipated, add expenses to this budget** **or remember to budget savings in addition to** **the cost of regular home maintenance.)**	**Monthly**	**Annual**
Rent/Mortgage payment		
Home/Household insurance		
Home maintenance		
Condo/Association monthly fees		
Property tax		
Telephone		
Electricity/Natural gas		
Water		

EXPENSES		
Auto loan/Lease payments		
Auto insurance		
Gasoline		
Food		
Healthcare and related insurance		
Employer provided group plan contribution		
Dental		
Medicare supplement		
Long-term care		
Disability		
Other		
Healthcare expense not covered by insurance		
Prescriptions		
Medical supplies		
Treatment co-pays		
Dental/vision/hearing		
Over-the-counter medications		

EXPENSES		
Medical transportation		
Life Insurance		
Child support		
Alimony		
Recreation and entertainment (hobbies, memberships, dining out, events [sports, movies, plays], other)		
Charitable donations and gifts		
Direct caregiving expenses (e.g., cost of in-home paid caregiver not covered by insurance, additional expenses associated with caring for a dependent/disabled child or other family member)		
Incidental caregiving expenses (e.g., gifts for facility staff at Christmas)		

EXPENSES		
Other (child care, college tuition and expenses, clothing, etc.)		
Total these expenses.		

Net Income—Subtract Total Expenses from Total Income	

Remember to attach any necessary documentation—inventory copies, copy of Safety/Security/Condition Checklist, etc.— to the completed Questionnaire.